Kitchen Sense for Disabled People

The Disabled Living Foundation would like to acknowledge the generous assistance of the Campbell Soup Company.

The Disabled Living Foundation would also like to thank the Home Service and the Public Relations Departments of British Gas for their donation towards the publication costs.

KITCHEN SENSE FOR DISABLED PEOPLE

Edited by Gwen Conacher FIHEc

Illustrations by Brenda Naylor

CROOM HELM
London • Sydney • Dover, New Hampshire
on behalf of the Disabled Living Foundation

Croom Helm Ltd, Provident House, Burrell Row,
Beckenham, Kent BR3 1AT

Croom Helm Australia Pty Ltd, Suite 4, 6th Floor,
64-76 Kippax Street, Surry Hills, NSW 2010, Australia

British Library Cataloguing in Publication Data

Kitchen sense for disabled people.
1. Home economics for the physically handicapped.
I. Conacher, Gwen II. Disabled Living Foundation
640'.240816 TX147

ISBN 0-7099-4512-4

Croom Helm, 51 Washington Street, Dover,
New Hampshire 03820, USA

Library of Congress Cataloging in Publication Data

Kitchen sense for disabled people
on behalf of the Disabled Living Foundation.
Bibliography: P.
Includes index.
1. Cookery for the physically handicapped.
2. Self-help devices for the disabled. I. Conacher, Gwen. II. Disabled living foundation.
TX652.K4685 1986 641.5'0240816 86-4500
ISBN 0-7099-4512-4 (PBK.)

Typeset in 10pt Times Roman by Leaper & Gard Ltd, Bristol, England
Printed and bound in Great Britain
by Billing & Sons Limited, Worcester.

Contents

List of Contributors
Members of the Steering Group
Foreword
Foreword to the Previous Edition
1. Kitchen Design *Jean Symons* 1
2. Equipment *Gwen Conacher* 22
3. Coping with Problems *Marian Lane* 56
4. Healthy Eating *Creina Murland* 106
5. Eating in Company *Gwen Conacher* 113
6. Shopping *Gwen Conacher* 118
7. Short Cuts in Cooking *Gwen Conacher* 127
Appendix I: Sources of Advice and Help 147
Appendix II: Addresses of Suppliers 152
Appendix III: Further Reading 156
Index 161

List of Contributors

Gwen Conacher, FIHEc, worked for Unilever Ltd from 1955 to 1966, first as a demonstrator, then as head of the Food and Cookery Centre Demonstration Service and finally as consumer research organiser of the Welwyn Research Laboratories. From 1966 to 1981 she was home economist to the Electricity Council. A founder member of the Institute of Home Economics, Mrs Conacher was the National Chairman from 1973 to 1975. She is the author of several books on food freezing.

Marian Lane, DipCOT, worked as an occupational therapist before joining the Disabled Living Foundation's Information Service in 1972. She became head of the Information Service in 1980 and, from 1983 to 1985, led the team working on the computerisation of the Information Bank. She was a co-author of the first version of this book, *Kitchen Sense for Disabled or Elderly People* (1977).

Creina Murland, SRD, is district dietitian for the Riverside Health Authority (Victoria Sector), London, and was chairman of the British Dietetic Association from 1972 to 1974. She has written numerous articles on dietetics for professional journals.

Jean Symons, AADipl RIBA, was from 1968 to 1971 assistant director of the Centre for Advanced Studies in Environment; from 1972 to 1981, consultant architect to the Centre on Environment for the Handicapped (CEH), London; and from 1974 to 1979, director of CEH. She was the Royal Institute of British Architects' representative on the committee which produced the British Standards on 'Design of Housing for the Convenience of Disabled People' 1978, and 'Access for the Disabled to Buildings' 1979. She is at present on the Kitchen Furniture and Domestic Appliances Technical Committee. Mrs Symons is the author of a number of design guides and articles on the needs of disabled people in public buildings and in the home.

Material on the needs of visually handicapped people throughout the book has been contributed by:

Valerie Scarr, FBCO, DCLP, DOrth, adviser on visual handicap for the Disabled Living Foundation since 1978. Previously she was senior ophthalmic optician, West of England Eye Infirmary, Exeter, and more recently contact lens practitioner, Moorfields Eye Hospital, London. Mrs Scarr has also worked in New Zealand as senior ophthalmic optician and orthoptist, Dunedin Hospital.

Margaret Ford, DipSocStudies CTB, an experienced social worker, who has contributed for 12 years to the BBC's weekly programme for visually handicapped people, *In Touch.* She is also joint author of the BBC's standard work of practical advice for visually handicapped people, also named *In Touch.*

Members of the Steering Group

Lady Hamilton, CBE MA, Chairman, Disabled Living Foundation.
Miss E. Fanshawe, OBE, DipCOT, Director, Disabled Living Foundation.
Miss S. Beazeley, DipCOT, Principal Occupational Therapist, Hammersmith and Fulham Social Services.
Miss L. Bradshaw, DipCOT, Head Research Occupational Therapist, The London Hospital.
S. Bradshaw, Director, Spinal Injuries Association.
Mrs E. Barrett, District Domiciliary Care Manager, South Westminster, London.
Miss Agnes Cameron, ALCM CertEd, Former Chairman, National Association for the Education of the Partially Sighted.
Mrs A. Davies, Author and broadcaster.
Miss H. Edwards, DipCOT, Former Information Officer, Disabled Living Foundation.
Mrs M. Ford, DipSocStudies CTB, Social Worker for the Visually Handicapped Elderly Person.
Mrs E. Grove, FCOT, Occupational Therapy Adviser, DHSS, London.
Mrs A. Hutt, SRN OHNC HVTutor RNT, Royal College of Nursing Society of Geriatric Nursing.
Mrs E. Lloyd, SROT, Disabled Living Adviser, Harrow Social Services.
Miss W. Matthews, MBE FIHEc MRSH, Home Service Adviser, British Gas Corporation.
Miss J. Ryan, DipCOT, Information Officer, Disabled Living Foundation.
Mrs V. Scarr, FBCO DCLP DOrth, Visual Handicap Adviser, Disabled Living Foundation.
Dr M.C. Stewart, MB BS DObstRCOG, Principal Medical Officer (Adult Health), Basingstoke and North Hampshire Health Authority.
Miss J. Sutherland, DipCOT SROT, Head Occupational Therapist, Victoria Health Authority, London.
Miss E.R. Wilshire, MCSP ONC MIInfSc, Compiler, Equipment for the Disabled (Mary Marlborough Lodge, Nuffield Orthopaedic Centre, Oxford).
Miss M. Wadhams, Former Skin Project Officer, Disabled Living Foundation.
J.H. Wyatt, JP DPA, General Secretary, Disabled Living Foundation.

Foreword

The problems of the disabled housewife have been known to the Disabled Living Foundation (DLF) for many years, almost since our work began. Our serious investigations began in 1966 when Miss Phyllis Howie, TDipCOT, conducted a pioneering survey, *A Pilot Study of Disabled Housewives in Their Kitchens*, in which the problems of the disabled housewife were studied and compared to those of a matched control group of able-bodied housewives. Since then, every study has confirmed the special needs of the disabled person responsible for running the home, whether man or woman. Numerous problems include inability to use kitchen storage, to make a hot meal, to see if equipment is dirty or to shop for food.

Our first textbook, *Kitchen Sense for Disabled or Elderly People*, was published in 1975 and reprinted in subsequent years. The work and study on which it was based were mostly undertaken in 1974 or earlier. Since then there have been changes; items of equipment which were uncommon in 1974 are now in common use, much new equipment has come on the market and the range and availability of convenience foods has greatly increased. The universal spread of supermarkets and the almost total disappearance of goods deliveries to the door have altered shopping habits. Again since 1974, the problems of visually handicapped people with enough useful residual vision to enable them to work in the kitchen have been explored and possible solutions found.

In short, to provide an up-to-date textbook a complete revision was necessary. This book is the result.

Some completely new aspects have been covered. The problems of people who do not see very well, not considered in the first edition, are now included. Assisted by the Royal National Institute for the Deaf, we have also covered some problems of deaf people. Since planning and design have developed and equipment has become more versatile, we invited an architect to contribute to this new edition.

The Campbell Soup Company of America generously funded the original *Kitchen Sense*. This Company agreed once again to fund both the research and the writing of what has proved, in the event, to be a new work. The Trustees of the Disabled Living Foundation thank the Campbell Soup Company very warmly for their continuing interest, which has extended to practical help and advice as well as finance. We feel exceptionally lucky that they have maintained their interest for nearly 12 years. The

Trustees are also very grateful to the Home Service and Public Relations Departments of British Gas for financial help towards the publication costs and also to members of its staff contributing to, and commenting on, the text. The DLF Trustees believe that the team which has jointly produced the book is of unusual calibre. In particular, we felt most fortunate in obtaining the services of Mrs G. Conacher, FIHEc, the Editor (and also a substantial contributor to the book), who has worked throughout as a volunteer. It has not been an easy book to prepare and the Trustees would like to express their gratitude to the authors, Miss Marian Lane, DipCOT, Miss Creina Murland, SRD, and Mrs Jean Symons, AADipl, RIBA, and also to Mrs Margaret Ford, DipSocStudies, CTB, and Mrs Valerie Scarr, FBCO, DCLP, DOrth, who made contributions on visual handicap throughout the book. They also thank Mrs Brenda Naylor, the DLF's illustrator, who has again provided the line drawings which add so much to the clarity, interest and persuasiveness of the book.

Sadly, Miss Sydney Foott, who wrote and edited the previous book and who would certainly have involved herself in the new version, died in 1978. The foundations laid by her and by her colleagues in that book, Miss Jill Mara, a home economist with a special interest in research, and Miss Marian Lane, who provided the occupational material, have been of great value in producing the new one. Fortunately, Miss Lane has continued her interest in the subject, and has contributed her knowledge and experience once more.

The work has been steered by an eminent advisory panel of experts who have each made their own contributions and have discussed, criticised and suggested points while the manuscript was being drafted. The DLF Trustees are most grateful to them for their help which has been most generously given.

We hope that the present work will prove useful not only to disabled people, by making their work easier and helping them to maintain their independence, but to those, whatever their discipline, who help them to manage in the kitchen.

Developments in kitchen planning, design and equipment, in food technology and in nutritional knowledge are continuing all the time. This book will therefore need revising from time to time and ultimately completely rewriting once again.

As ever, the DLF will greatly welcome comments, criticisms and further information, so that when the next edition is written it can be made truly useful.

W.M. Hamilton
Chairman
Disabled Living Foundation

Foreword to the Previous Edition*

The Disabled Living Foundation has been interested in the disabled housewife of all ages for many years. Every investigation confirmed our belief in her — or his — problems, for it must be remembered that many disabled housewives are male. The problems ranged from inability to use any of the storage in the kitchen to inability even to get a hot meal. The members of the DLF's Advisory Panel on Equipment (under whose auspices this book is written and to whom the DLF Trustees are much indebted) were engaged in preliminary work on a cookbook for disabled people when 'Mealtime Manual' was published in the USA. One of us was asked to review it and having seen the content of this admirable book — unfortunately largely unusable in this country because of different equipment, foods, climate and eating habits — we immediately raised our sights. We wrote to Campbells in America supported by our friend, Sir Roy Matthews, one time Chairman of Crosse and Blackwell Ltd, who spoke for us to the then President of the Campbell Soup Company, Mr W.B. Murphy, who himself also took a personal interest in our project. We met the Managing Director of Campbells Soups Ltd (the English company), Mr H. Kitching, and after very short explanations we received our grant. The DLF Trustees thank these gentlemen warmly. Without them, and without the generosity of the Campbell Soup Company, we could not have attempted a project on this scale.

Our next piece of good fortune lay in persuading Miss Sydney Foott to undertake the writing of the book, and in finding her colleagues, Miss Lane and Miss Mara. They were hard and enthusiastic workers, and the DLF has never had a better team. We enrolled a working party, from the Panel and others, to advise in detail, and through giving the project a great deal of publicity at the commencement received the practical suggestions of many disabled people.

The Campbell Soup Company most kindly sent their Home Economist, Miss Claire Boasi, to visit London to help us, and large consignments of helpful equipment for our consideration. Dr Rusk and Mrs Klinger from the Institute of Rehabilitation Medicine, New York University, offered all possible co-operation. To all our advisers, whether individuals or organisations, we are deeply grateful.

---

*Published as *Kitchen Sense for Disabled or Elderly People*, by S. Foott, M. Lane and J. Mara (Heinemann Health Books for the Disabled Living Foundation, 1977, revised edition).

Foreword

Now that the book is written, Campbells Soups Ltd have offered most welcome financial help in launching it, which will enable us to give more review copies and more publicity in an attempt to reach the very large numbers of people whom it could help.

It is rare that a single person can by himself assist such a large group of people as the disabled. Such attempts as this book involve very many people and a great deal of pioneering practical work. The DLF Trustees thank all the people who helped. Our great hope now is that the users of the book, whoever they may be, will criticise and make suggestions so that if Miss Foott agrees, as we trust she will, to revise it for a second edition, she can make it more comprehensive and more useful. Therefore in expressing our gratitude to the generous helpers of the past, may we ask readers to send in their comments and invite their help for the future?

W.M. Hamilton
Chairman
Disabled Living Foundation

1 Kitchen Design

Jean Symons

'When a kitchen is well planned, then it is easier for able-bodied and disabled housewives alike.' So began the original edition of *Kitchen Sense.* Possibly the greatest changes since then are the increased awareness of the abilities of people with disabilities, the recognition that the person responsible for running the home is less certain to be female and the increasing versatility of kitchen fittings.

Properly designed, a kitchen can overcome many of the difficulties of the disabled user. Increasingly, kitchens and kitchen equipment are being designed for elderly people and wheelchair users. Advice is available to the architects engaged in such purpose-built housing and to the designers and manufacturers of kitchen equipment for 'mobility' and 'wheelchair' use about the general assumptions on which their designs should be based. Purpose-built designs of this kind will help to overcome many difficulties and limitations of the users for whom they are intended. The results may not always be ideal for the specific problems of individual users. This chapter is not about the technical guidance which is available to professionals who are designing housing for disabled people in general. It is for people who have physical disabilities and wish to make the right decisions to overcome their specific individual problems so that they can be as independent as possible (even if there are people using the kitchen who are not disabled).

People do not necessarily move their home as they become older, more frail or handicapped; they may need to make modifications to help them remain where they are. A British Standard Code of Practice for *Design of Housing for the Convenience of Disabled People* (BS 5619: 1978) describes the provision which should be made in ordinary new housing to enable this to happen. The specific recommendations on 'Kitchens' are discussed later (see p. 3).

Much will depend on the money available. Severely disabled people who live in some local authority areas may be able to obtain a grant enabling them to have a kitchen designed specifically for them which will be envied by all their friends and neighbours.

Even without such resources, many difficulties of disabled and elderly people can be resolved or mitigated by planning a kitchen to meet their individual needs and carefully selecting well designed fittings and equipment.

Kitchen Users — People

People may be tall, short, fat or thin; unable to reach high or to bend low; have difficulty lifting heavy pans, reading labels or even seeing where they have put things down; some cannot stand up and others cannot easily sit down; some cannot hear and others have to cope with allergic reactions including skin conditions. But everybody needs to eat and therefore to prepare food — or have it prepared for them.

In 1980 the London Borough of Hillingdon Social Services published *Clients' Opinions of Wheelchair Housing* based on interviews with 49 tenants who had moved into *purpose designed* wheelchair housing. It was reported that 20 tenants found it difficult or impossible to reach their kitchen storage (and work surfaces) because cupboards were too high, too low or too deep for them, several mentioned lack of space for fridges and washing machines, 35 had difficulty opening some of their windows and 25 had difficulty in operating heating controls.

This shows how important it is to consider, whenever possible, the needs of individual users. Many of the difficulties can be overcome and some solutions are discussed in this chapter and in Chapter 2.

Development of Kitchens

When adapting older kitchens, it is important to understand how kitchen design has developed during the last 40 years. Before 1939, when the Second World War began, little consideration had been given to the design of kitchens — they had just evolved. By 1945, when the war ended after a period with almost no domestic building, guidelines were being drawn up incorporating many ideas adopted from other countries (mainly the USA and Sweden). This led to the development of the fitted kitchen and the acceptance of the need for standard sizes and dimensions to accommodate sink, cooker and fridge, so that the aim of continuous worktops could be achieved. In addition, the availability of refrigerators contributed to the reduction in the size of larders and ultimately to their virtual disappearance.

The introduction of other equipment such as dishwashers, clothes-washers and dryers, freezers, mixers, split-level cookers and rotisseries are dealt with in Chapter 2.

Until recently, the cooker was a self-contained piece of equipment, for which a suitable space had to be left; the sink, combined with integral draining boards, was fitted on top of a standard kitchen unit. However, many people found it difficult to reach the standard units, especially those in wheelchairs for whom they were not only too high but also inaccessible because of the cupboard unit supporting them. This led to the design of special units to satisfy the needs of people in wheelchairs (see p. 8).

In recent years there has been a basic change in the design of kitchens which can benefit people who cannot use the old standard units. Both sinks and cooker hobs can be built into holes in the worktop which can be fixed at any height, according to the client's requirements — if he or she foregoes the standard cupboards underneath.

Looking to the future, the greater flexibility needed to accommodate individual choice may foreshadow a time when there will be less emphasis on built-in units. Kitchen users are likely to require freedom to decide what they want in their kitchen; cheaper worktops, which could be replaced if needs change (for instance, new sink or cooker hob unit), combined with adjustable shelves, may need to be considered.

The most recent guidance in *Homes for the Future* (1983) is: 'It is likely that in future an average kitchen will need to accommodate a split-level oven and hob, a large refrigerator, a deep-freeze cabinet, a dishwasher, a washing machine and a tumble dryer. Variations in the shape and size of such appliances must be allowed for in the kitchen layout. With this in mind, an increase in floor space and a reduction in the number of built-in cupboards would seem to be justified — particularly if there is enclosed general storage space at ground floor level near to the kitchen.' It also recommends that worktop/units should not be positioned under kitchen windows.

Formerly, it was positively recommended that the sink should be underneath the kitchen window for good lighting and so that the washer-up could look outside. Those considerations may still be persuasive and the layout of an existing kitchen may be difficult to change. Such a layout has its disadvantages, however: the window is difficult to open, particularly for disabled people, it gets splashed and is hard to clean. The modern guidance is that windows should, if possible, not be over sinks and worktops. But there are still people who want their sink under the kitchen window!

The Government Role

British Standard Recommendations

The British Standard on the *Design of Housing for the Convenience of Disabled People* (BS 5619: 1978) makes recommendations about design which should be included in ordinary housing if it is to be convenient for disabled people to live in or visit. Its suggestions might make it possible for people who became disabled to remain in their own home. The section on kitchens recommends:

1. kitchen planning: A continuous sequence of units is recommended, comprising worktop/sink/worktop/cooker/worktop (see p. 7);
2. floor space: There should be unobstructed floor space in kitchens to allow for wheelchair manoeuvre. The minimum clear space should be

1,400 × 1,400 mm (approx. 55 × 55 in);
3. kitchen dining facilities: Provision should be made for meals to be taken in the kitchen area. Where the dining room is separate from the kitchen, there should be adequate space inside the kitchen for two people to take meals;
4. kitchen units (it is to be remembered that this is advice for ordinary, good design).

Dimensions — worktops should be at 900 mm (approx. 36 in) above floor level.

Working arrangements — provision should be made to enable work in the kitchen to be done from a seated position. The incorporation of pull-out boards below the fixed work surface is suggested.

Storage — as much storage accommodation as possible should be at levels that can comfortably be reached. Storage shelves in general use should not be higher than 1,600 mm (63 in) above floor level.

Sinks — sink bowls should be relatively shallow. A bowl depth of 150 mm (6 in) is suggested and a domestic type lever-action swivel mixer sink tap is recommended in order to permit pans and kettles to be placed on an adjacent surface for filling.

The British Standard also mentions that floor surfaces should be slip-resistant, that refuse disposal facilities be easily accessible and that consideration should be given to the specification of windows in relation to safety, accessibility of controls and cleaning.

Wheelchair and Mobility Housing

Most of the recommendations on kitchens made by Goldsmith in *Mobility Housing* (1974) were included in BS 5619 (see p. 3); the relevant points from *Wheelchair Housing* (1975) (also by Goldsmith) are covered in the following pages.

The Department of the Environment circular *Adaptations of Housing for People Who are Physically Handicapped* (1978) lists all the things a disabled person *should* be entitled to have done, either through the local authority or the Department of Health and Social Security (DHSS). Ask a local authority occupational therapist or one at the hospital you are attending for advice on this.

Getting Financial Help

Adapting an existing kitchen or having a new one fitted can be an expensive business. Anyone registered as disabled with the local social services department may well be entitled to financial help in the form of a local authority improvement grant or a social services grant. Improvement grants can also be obtained to bring kitchens up to minimum space standards, and for the first-time supply of essential materials. 'First time' is sometimes interpreted quite literally if a new item is installed to replace existing equipment which the kitchen user could not reach. Contact the local social services department; the occupational therapist should be able to help with the decision-making and designing, and also outline the procedures involved in getting financial help. When a local authority does not employ an occupational therapist, the housing department's grants officer will make an assessment of grant. It is most important not to start the work before any grant application has been approved because grants, except in very rare cases, cannot be paid retrospectively.

Some charities offer financial help; the social worker or occupational therapist should be able to advise on details of local charities.

Making Your Plans (Layout)

The suggestions which follow are not exhaustive nor will they apply to everyone. The aim is to help you to decide how best to attain what is best for you — given your constraints (physical or financial), your preferences and your way of life.

To achieve the result which is most likely to satisfy your specific requirements, list the activities which you and others want to carry out in the kitchen, either because it is the obvious place or because there is nowhere else. Having made your list, measured your kitchen and counted your money, it will be easier to make decisions; you will probably also have to make some compromises.

Some people use their kitchen as a living room, others regard it as a workshop. Some are the sole user, in which case most things should be accessible. People in wheelchairs need more space to manoeuvre than those with walking difficulties who might need to support themselves on the nearest object (which must, therefore, be stable). However, if accessibility means sacrificing potential storage space (for instance, shelves which you cannot reach but someone else could) consider carefully before deciding not to have shelves above a height prescribed in design guidance for disabled people (see p. 4).

Look at as many kitchens as you can, talk to friends and advisers, visit an aids centre, study books and magazines and send for brochures (or visit showrooms if you can). Kitchens are expensive, so do not be pressurised by kitchen sales people but make sure you get what you want or need; manufacturers are sometimes prepared to help with a specific request (for instance, an individually designed trolley or non-standard pieces). (See also Chapter 3).

Most of the kitchens being considered by readers are likely to be adaptations either of existing kitchens or of a space where it is proposed to construct a kitchen. Some are large enough to accommodate all the equipment chosen in the ideal position, others are so small that they are virtually a cupboard (Figure 1.1).

Figure 1.1: Compact Kitchen Developed by the Institute of Rehabilitation Medicine, New York

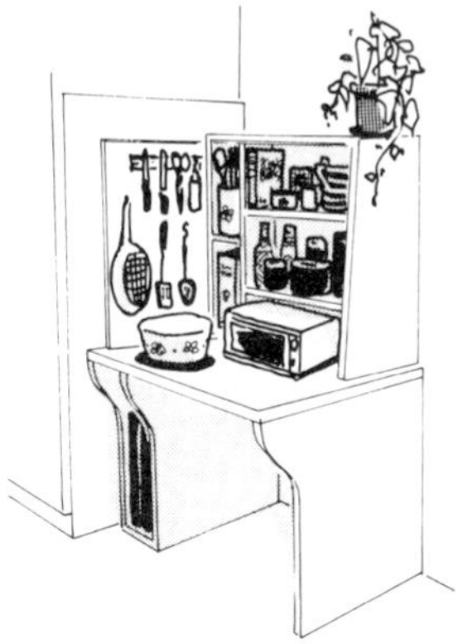

Whatever their size, most kitchens *will* have: a sink (or two); a cooker (or, to be more correct, a hob, grill, oven or oven/grill); worktop/preparation space; storage space; lighting (natural/electric); ventilation; water supply and other services. Many kitchens *may* have: more sophisticated storage space (fridges and freezers); a variety of cooking facilities; waste disposal unit; clothes washer and dryer; dishwasher; table, chairs, stools, trolleys and other freestanding furniture.

If possible, draw a plan of your kitchen to scale on squared grid paper with all the doors, windows, hatches, built-in equipment and services marked in. Then draw in all movable equipment (remembering door openings and overhangs) again to scale and see where it best fits into the plan. (If necessary, make an elevation to take account of heights.) Alternatively, cut squares of card to correct size to represent the major appliances and furniture (tables, chairs and so on) and move them around on the plan until the best arrangement is found (Figure 1.2).

It is worth considering a hatch to the dining room for people who have difficulty walking. Remember that doors can be removed at little cost, and that refrigerators can be moved quite easily so long as there is a suitable power point, whereas cookers are more expensive to move as this may entail new connections by the gas or electricity board.

If you are adapting an old kitchen with units dating from the 1940s or 1950s, bear in mind that the standard measurement was then 3 ft × 1 ft 9 in × 1 ft 9 in, 3 ft 6 in or 5 ft 3 in, so that new equipment with metric dimensions will not 'line up' with the old units.

When planning the placing of individual items also take into account your work sequence (usually: storage, preparation, cooking, serving, eating, washing up, storage) which may strengthen your decision to have a door or cupboard moved so that it does not interfere with the efficient preparation of food (Figure 1.3).

Figure 1.2: Kitchen Plans: Based on Examples of Standard Plans (Goldsmith, 1984, 3rd edn, revised) (a) Corridor Layout; (b) L-Layout; (c) U-Layout

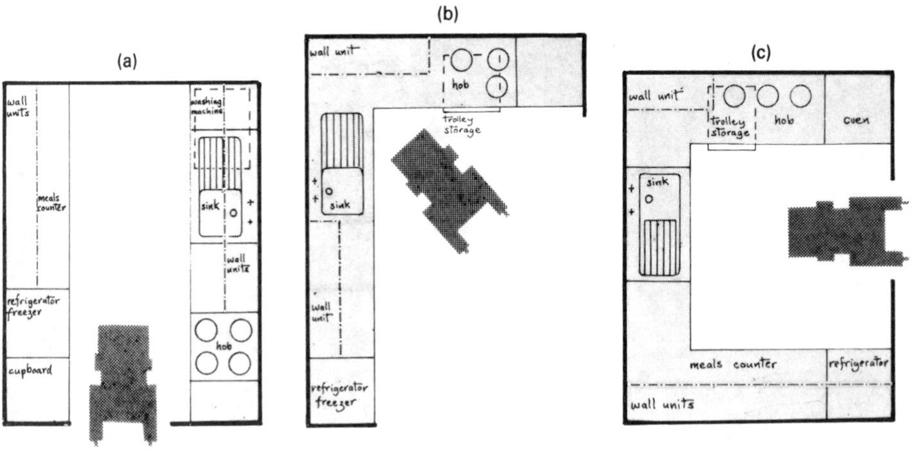

Figure 1.3: Work Sequence in Kitchen

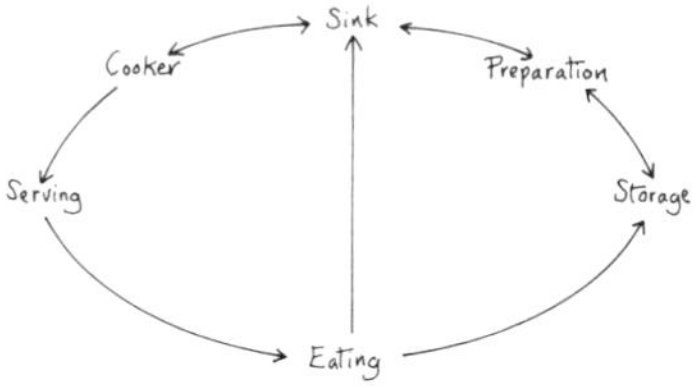

Also, bear in mind the relative frequency of your movements between fixed working areas in the kitchen (Figure 1.4) which shows that disabled users move most frequently between the sink and the cooker, and that they move more frequently than able-bodied users between the sink and the dining table since they can carry articles only singly, or in small quantities.

It may be a long time before your decisions about alterations are put into practice, so consider how to cope while the work is being done, as builders cannot avoid making a mess or at least causing disruption.

What Fittings Should You Choose?

Kitchen Units — Standard Dimensions

A new British Standard (BS 6222: Part 1, 1982) aims to co-ordinate the dimensions of kitchen equipment — kitchen units (fitments) and appliances (Figure 1.5). Manufacturers should be using these dimensions and, in

Figure 1.4: Relative Frequency of Movements between Fixed Working Areas of Kitchen (Illustrating P.M. Howie's Findings in *A Pilot Study of Disabled Housewives in Their Kitchens*)

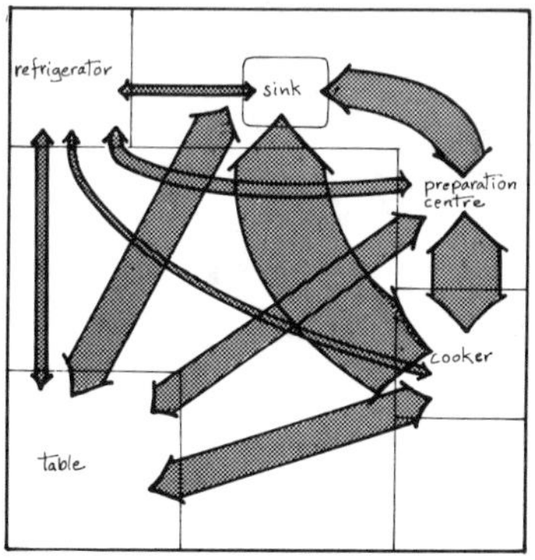

Source: Goldsmith, s. (1984) *Designing for the Disabled,* 3rd edn (revised), RIBA Publications, London

Figure 1.5: Kitchen Units: Standard Terms and Dimensions

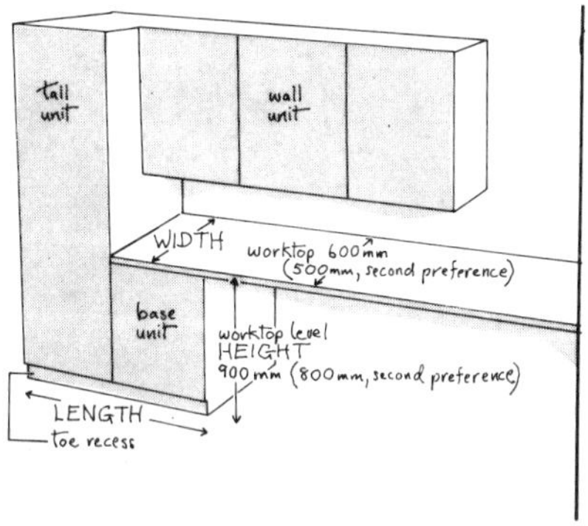

Based on BS 6222: Part 1, 1982

theory, any appliance should fit any make of unit. But be warned: publications and catalogues often confuse the terms 'width', 'depth', 'breadth' and 'length', so before ordering anything, check that you and the suppliers are discussing the same dimension.

The BS definition of length is logically remembered as 'length along wall'. Width is from front to back, which means that most worktops are 600 mm (approx. 24 in) *wide.* The definition of height remains unchanged. (Some manufacturers use the British Standard measurement referred to as 'second preference' for units especially designed for people with limited reach, but this is really designed for housing where the tenant is unknown, whereas this book is about individual choice).

Decide which kind of sink, taps, worktop and storage space (which may or may not be built into standard kitchen units) are best for the person(s) using the kitchen (in the same way that you choose appliances and aids, if necessary seek advice from an occupational therapist). If the answer is a series of built-in units, then some of these are very well designed for people with special needs (Figure 1.6a and b), but if the answer is a range of adjustable open shelves and adjustable units, that is equally acceptable (Figure 1.7a and b).

It is no longer necessary to fit everything along the kitchen walls. People with very large kitchens could consider the more expensive alternative of installing an island unit containing a cooker and a sink.

Figure 1.6a: Homat Purpose-designed Kitchen

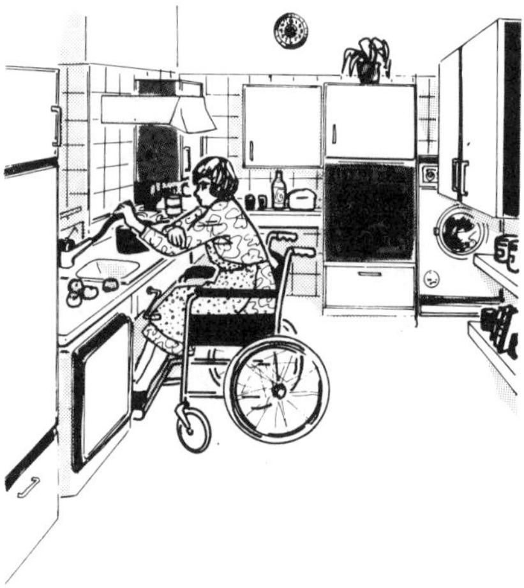

Figure 1.6b: Kitchen Units Designed for Wheelchair Housing

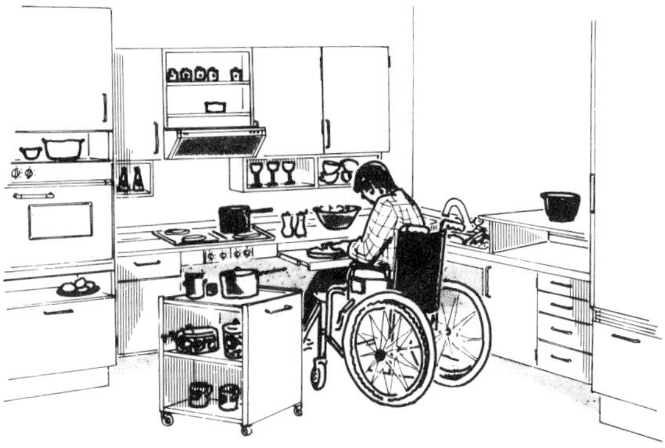

Figure 1.7a: Adjustable Shelves

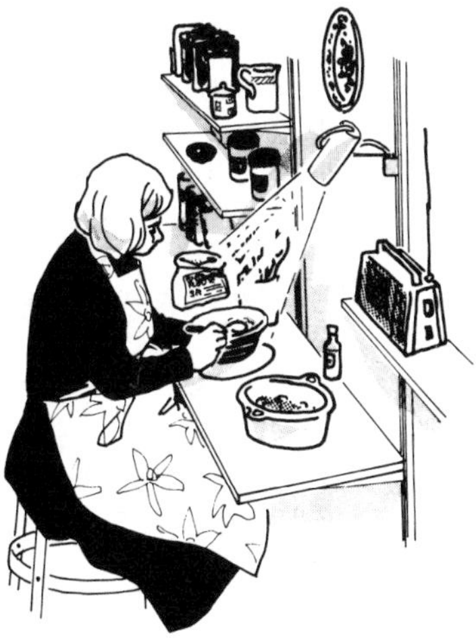

Figure 1.7b: Adjustable Wall Unit

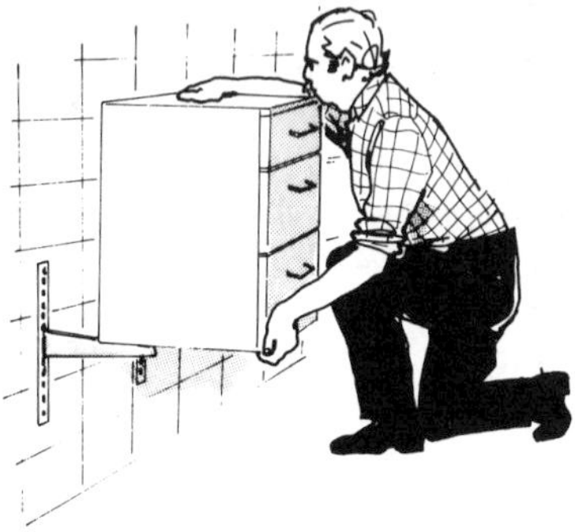

Figure 1.8a: Sink Moulded with Worktop (Corian)

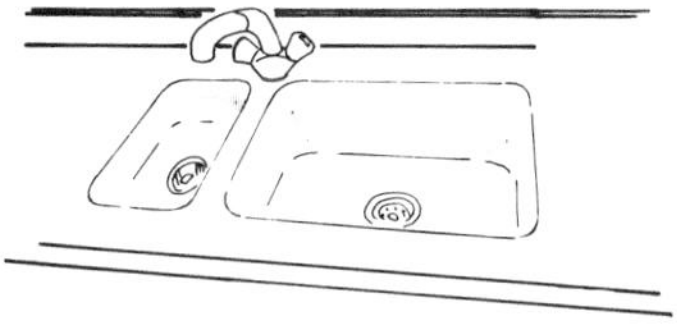

Figure 1.8b: One of a Large Selection of Drop-in Sinks

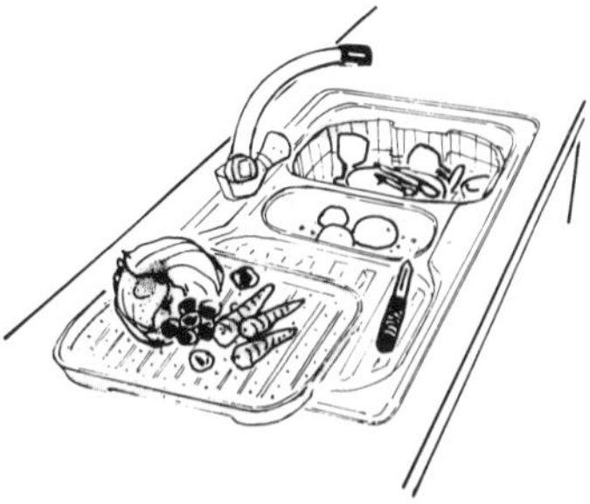

Sinks

Sinks, now available in many shapes, colours and sizes, are no longer restricted to the dimensions of the base units which support them. They can be obtained to include a variety of boards, drainers, strainers and bowls (Figure 1.8a), and can be moulded with the work surface (Figure 1.8b).

Draining boards can be integral or the adjacent worktop can be used — the surface and edge detailing should take this into consideration (see p. 13).

The recommended internal depth for wheelchair users (where the client is unknown) is 130–140 mm (approx. 5–5.5 in) (see Figure 3.22); whereas the depth for other people ranges from 140 to 180 mm (approx. 5.5 to 7 in) or more. However, for a wheelchair user, this measurement will be influenced by the type of wheelchair used. Some smaller sinks do not have any overflow outlet, which can be a hazard. Many chairs have detachable armrests, while the interchangeable desk-type armrest enables the disabled person to get closer to the sink or work surface.

Space permitting, you should consider whether to have two sinks at different heights if joint users of the kitchen find the other's ideal unacceptable. It should not be necessary to compromise at a level which suits neither.

Adjustable sinks are available, but remember that the height is difficult to alter once the sink has been installed and that they are expensive.

Plumbing should be kept as far back and as neat as possible. If it is exposed, a panel forming a duct under the work surface could prevent dirt traps and improve the appearance.

Consider whether you need a waste disposal unit (this can also get in the way of a wheelchair user's knees).

If someone has no temperature sensation or is likely to damage sensitive skin by knocking it, the bottom of the sink and pipes should be insulated. The siting of the sink is discussed on page 3. If it is not possible to find an alternative to placing the sink under the window, consider how the window can be opened (see p. 19).

Taps

There is a large range of taps, but lever taps are the easiest to turn (Figure 1.9a). Points to consider when choosing taps include:

1. a tap turner used with existing taps (see Chapter 3, page 86);
2. a high-necked swivel mixer makes it easier to fill pans and kettles (Figure 1.9a);
3. taps can be positioned to the side of the sink to make this easier, although such taps could interfere with the worktop/sink/drainer sequence;
4. press-down or toggle action taps possibly combined with a spray (Figure 1.9b);

Figure 1.9a: Lever-operated Taps and High-necked Swivel Outlet

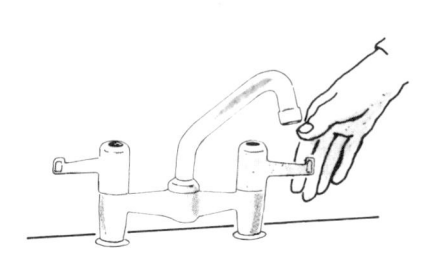

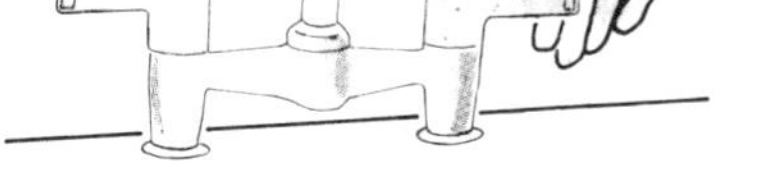

Figure 1.9b: Toggle Action Tap

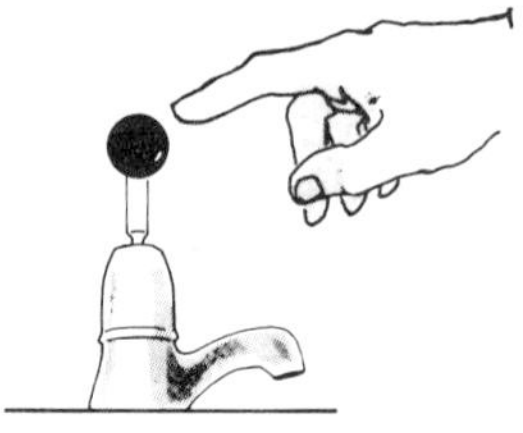

Figure 1.9c: Electronic Tap Operated by Putting Object Underneath

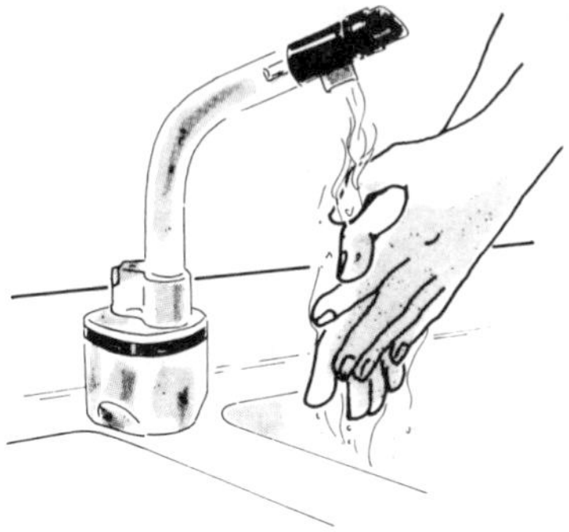

5. for people who cannot reach, controls can be mounted on the front of the worktop (and even controlled electrically).

It is also possible to buy the more expensive electronic taps which operate automatically if the hands (or an object) are placed under the tap (Figure 1.9c).

Worktops

Worktops can be cut to take the sink and hob unit of your choice. British Standard worktops are either 600mm or 500mm (approx. 24 or 20in, second preference) *wide* (front to back). Due to the fact that kitchen appliances are manufactured to standard sizes, the width needs to be 600mm (approx. 24in) to achieve a continuous line.

The height of a worktop is given as either 900mm or 850mm (approx. 36 or 34in, second preference). However, when considering your personal requirements, think whether your needs are likely to vary — for example, if your disability gets worse, it may be necessary to adjust the height of your worktop once it is installed.

It is possible to obtain adjustable fittings, but this type of expensive installation is more likely to be useful at assessment centres (so that people can experiment to find out which height will suit them best at home) rather than in the individually planned kitchen (this also applies to sinks, see p. 9). These fittings can be useful in houses that may be used by a succession of tenants.

People confined to wheelchairs or who are of restricted growth are likely to need a lower worktop with the result that fewer appliances will fit under the top. (See further discussion on storage, p. 14.)

In some households, the main kitchen user will not be the disabled person, so standard design is appropriate. However, it is useful to have a work

Figure 1.10: Upstand on Worktop

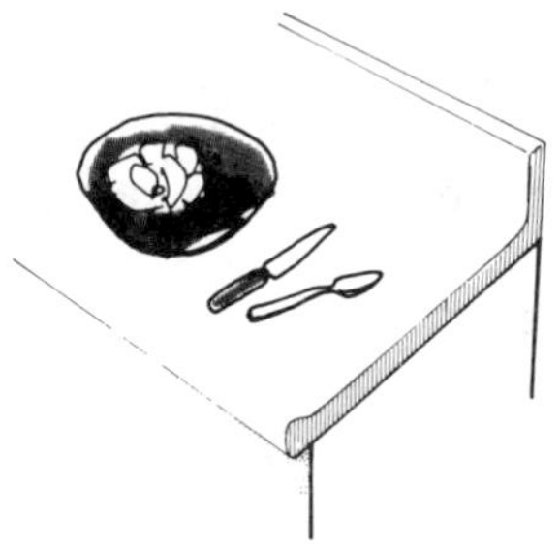

surface at a lower height for the wheelchair user so that he or she can make snacks.

Pull-out boards are useful to provide a lower height for some jobs and often include a hole to help stabilize mixing bowls. But make sure they cannot pull right out unintentionally. Pull-out surfaces are not suited to taking kettles or other electric appliances unless specifically designed to do so.

Finishes can be applied to existing units and edged with hardwood. This solution might help someone whose sight is failing by providing either less glare or more contrast.

Newer materials are often manufactured to incorporate an upstand at the back (Figure 1.10) and a raised, shaped front edge (to stop things sliding off and avoid sharp edges). They can also be cut or moulded to the user's specification. There is a large choice. Choose a rounded edge if your skin is delicate and easily damaged by knocks. Curved corners make cleaning easier.

If the draining board is not an integral part of the sink, choose the material carefully. Slip-resistant surfaces are now available and a recent, but expensive, development (Corian) can be formed to any shape (even to include sink bowls) (see Figure 1.8a); it is warm to touch, easy to clean, virtually unscratchable and rather expensive (but possibly worth it). See Appendix II, p. 153.

Cookers

Cookers are fully discussed in Chapter 2. However, when planning a kitchen, it must be remembered that, since the majority of cookers are now manufactured to fit in with standard kitchen units, the hob on a free-standing cooker is likely to be at 900 mm (approx. 36 in) with the oven below. Therefore, most wheelchair users or those who have difficulty bending will prefer, space permitting, separate hobs and oven units.

Storage

What do you want to store? The priorities of a dedicated cook will differ from those of someone who regards cooking as a necessary chore. Few people now have larders. These have been replaced by fridges, freezers and, sometimes, by a small (ventilated) store cupboard. Larders were used to store not only food but also larger items of less often used kitchen equipment, which are now generally stored at the back of low level kitchen cupboards — inaccessible to everyone.

Obviously, the most frequently used implements should be within easy reach. Storage systems which were originally designed for people with physical handicaps were among the first to incorporate shelves on cupboard doors (Figure 1.11), pull-out trays instead of drawers and shelves, and swivel trays in corner storage units. These useful details are now incorporated in many designs.

However, given that the fridge, freezer, cooker, washing machine, tumble dryer and/or dishwasher may occupy available floor space, a small kitchen will have little space for low-level, built-in cupboards ('base units').

Cupboards fixed some distance above the worktops ('wall units') — recommended height from floor to underside 1,300 mm (approx. 51 in) — are not useful to people in wheelchairs since they cannot reach above the bottom shelf (see Figure 1.5). However, as worktops are likely to be 600 mm (approx. 24 in) from front to back to accommodate standard appliances, the space at the back between the worktop and the underside of the cupboard should be fully utilised as it is particularly valuable for people with limited reach and limited vision.

Ideas to consider for that space are:

1. hanging utensils on hooks fixed to a batten;

Figure 1.11: Storage Space on Cupboard Door

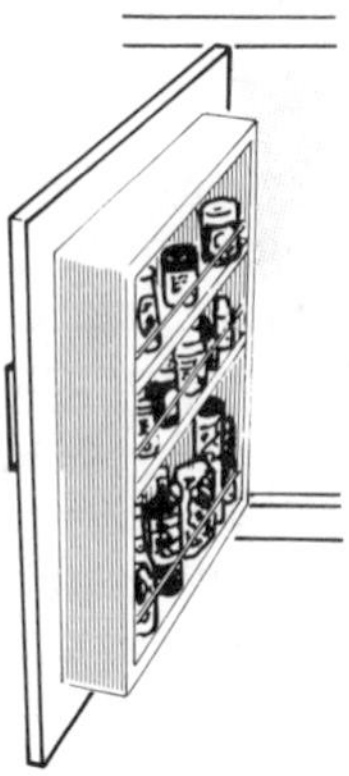

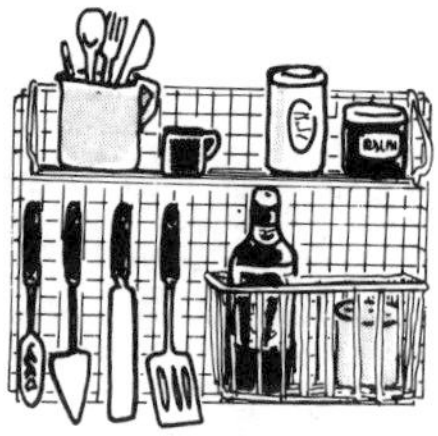

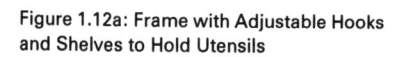

Figure 1.12a: Frame with Adjustable Hooks and Shelves to Hold Utensils

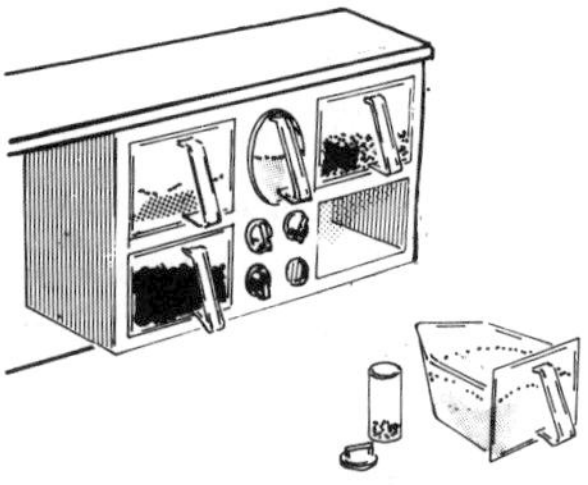

Figure 1.12b: Storage Boxes

2. traditional pegboard or newer plastic covered wire frames on which hooks, shelves and baskets can be hung (Figure 1.12a);
3. narrow glass-fronted cupboard with sliding doors and adjustable shelves;
4. narrow shelves on adjustable brackets;
5. storage boxes, made for tools and office use (Figure 1.12b).

If not used for shelves or cupboards, this space could provide a practical place to store small electrical appliances which are in frequent use.

Many consider that a range of shelves fixed along a wall are an excellent idea. Once the supports are fixed, shelves can be raised or lowered, their length and width changed and even light fittings and switches incorporated into some makes of uprights. A wider shelf at a convenient height can replace a table (especially in a confined space) for wheelchair users or others to sit at to work or eat (see Figure 1.7a). Supports and brackets are now available in many bright colours.

It is important to remember that shelves in a kitchen used by a visually handicapped person should be carefully sited so that they do not form an obstruction.

The storage space you need will depend on what you have to store in the kitchen, probably because there is no alternative. Even people who live alone and may not be able to reach, should think seriously before abandoning the idea of using space which is otherwise going to be wasted. Most people have visitors who will reach or climb up to get something. The main thing is to remember where it is stored and, if possible, anticipate the need. Some guidelines suggest that high-level space which the occupier cannot reach should be sealed off. This could prove frustrating.

It is important to consider details such as the type of cupboard doors, how drawers are divided and to try out handles and catches. Some people cannot pull horizontal handles, others cannot grip vertical handles, others prefer magnetic touch latches, and not many like knobs. Door furniture is available in many bright colours which could be helpful to those who cannot see well.

Sliding doors get in the way less than hinged doors (this is especially important for blind people), but the tracks are sometimes difficult to clean and, unless they are of good quality and run smoothly, can cause difficulties.

In existing kitchens, cupboard doors can be removed and be replaced by curtains or top-hung folding doors to hide under-sink chaos. This idea could be useful when modifying a kitchen for someone with restricted growth. If a false floor is installed, the cupboard doors removed and replaced as above, this will avert the expense of lowering the units and adapting the plumbing.

Drawers, pull-out shelves and storage baskets must glide smoothly and stops are essential to prevent them from pulling out too far.

The various kinds of trolleys (including mobile storage units and vegetable racks) used by many disabled and elderly people can be stored under the worktop and moved out easily when required.

When planning storage space, remember that other pieces of furniture, such as stools, chairs and waste bins, may need to be pushed under the worktop.

Finishes

Finishes are a matter of personal preference, and the points mentioned in this section remind readers of the special considerations they may need to think about.

Walls and Ceilings

The main problem is condensation, particularly if it is difficult to open and shut windows. Condensation may be worse in a bungalow as it is a single-storey building and it would be worthwhile insulating the kitchen (and other) ceiling(s), as well as external walls.

When choosing paint, make sure that it is washable (most modern paints are), and remember that, for visually handicapped people, contrasting colours on different surfaces often aid identification, while a very glossy paint causes too bright a reflection.

Floors

Floor finishes should be slip-resistant (when wet as well as dry) and skid-proof (which may depend as much on shoes as the floor surface). There is disagreement as to whether carpets in kitchens are practical or not, but some people (especially those with painful feet) may find that a carpet (preferably one that is easily cleaned) makes working in the kitchen more tolerable.

People who do not see well prefer a light, plain coloured floor rather than a patterned one so that they can detect things they have dropped. A contrasting coloured tile or strip can be installed in front of danger areas like the cooker.

Cork and linoleum in sheet or tile form are still popular and new materials are being developed all the time. Look at magazines and in shops, and consult the Disabled Living Foundation about those with suitable properties for your specific needs.

How to Run the Kitchen

The specific planning requirements for people with physical disabilities would benefit everyone: mains switches and stopcocks should be easy to reach, meters should be sited so that they can be read from outside the premises, and circuit breakers (the modern form of fuse box) should be easily accessible.

If the gas or electricity meter is inconveniently sited, contact the appropriate board and ask if the meter can be moved. It will only be possible to move it a short distance and there may be a charge for this service.

It is also worth considering whether to have a telephone socket in the kitchen.

Those who use solid fuel or LPG cylinders should remember that storage space will be necessary.

Gas

Gas may be used for heating and cooking. Whereas heating boilers and large multipoint heaters require flues, gas cookers and some small water heaters may not — but they do need good ventilation. Flexible hoses are available to enable freestanding gas cookers to be moved for cleaning.

British Gas has a team of home service advisers who will call on anyone at home and give free advice. All employees carry an identity card and a password can be arranged with blind customers (see also Chapter 2, p. 34).

People who are registered disabled or over 65 years and live alone qualify for free gas safety checks, including minor repairs. Modifications which can be made to appliances are mentioned in Chapter 2.

Water Supply

In the case of a completely redesigned or new kitchen, it is worth considering all the appliances which might be needed (even at a later date) when new plumbing is being installed — for instance, sink, waste disposal unit, washing machine, dishwasher, water heater, water softener — as it may be cheaper to make provision for future equipment than to make expensive adaptations later.

But heed the warning that some imported fittings which appear to be potentially useful are designed to work off high pressure systems and may not comply with British Water Board regulations. More important, they may not work efficiently, particularly in bungalows. If in doubt, contact the local water board for information.

Electricity

At least four dual socket outlets should be provided in the kitchen near the work surface, plus two for general use (see *Homes for the Future*). The Electricity Council (*Planning your Electric Kitchen*) recommends not less than four double sockets at worktop level in addition to the outlets for major appliances. There should also be a 30 amp cooker point.

Remember that trailing flexes can be dangerous. A recent development is 'track' conduit giving multiple outlets at regular intervals. It could be fixed in a convenient position for any user.

Of particular interest to people with visual difficulties are the plugs, sockets and cables in bright primary colours.

Remember that socket outlets should not be near a water supply. If an electric sink water heater is installed, it should be fitted by an electrician to a spur outlet.

The wiring regulations (IEE Wiring Regulations: Regulations for Electrical Installations*) contain the principles of good practice with which electricians should comply. All electric wiring installations should be carried out by a qualified electrician.

Any disabled person who needs advice should contact his or her area electricity board (under 'Electricity' in the telephone directory) and ask for someone to visit.

Plugs with handles and handles for plugs are available (see Chapter 3, p. 88); in addition, foot-operated, remote control and computer-operated switches are being developed.

Lighting

General Background Lighting

In a very small kitchen, a central overhead light may be sufficient to light the whole kitchen but, if possible, try to ensure that each centre of activity

* Issued by the Institute of Electrical Engineers, 15th edn, 1981.

has as much natural light as possible and its own lighting source. Fluorescent light (de luxe warm white for preference) gives less shadow, uses less electricity and the tubes last longer than tungsten bulbs.

Work Surface or Task Lighting

This is best provided by fixing strip lighting to the front underside of wall cupboards or shelves above the work surface. If this is not possible, lights should be fixed to the wall or ceiling over the work area. Glare (from light reflected from shiny surfaces) should be avoided; one way of achieving this is to fit a dimmer switch so that each person using the area can adjust the light. Contrasting colours are especially beneficial for people with bad sight (see Finishes, p. 16).

Heating

A wall-mounted fan heater is ideal in old kitchens to give comfort and prevent condensation, but remember that the control switch must be within easy reach. In newer kitchens, it is recommended (*Homes for the Future*) that elderly and disabled people need a uniform temperature throughout their homes of not less than 21°C; the suggested temperature for most kitchens is 16°C minimum.

Ventilation

Disabled and elderly people may find it difficult to open and close windows, particularly if they have to reach across a worktop.

Various window-opening devices are available, operated either electrically or by a lightweight, easy-grip extension handle. It might be worth considering replacing the existing window with one that slides.

An alternative form of ventilation is essential to prevent an accumulation of cooking smells and to prevent condensation (especially for people who have difficulty opening windows).

Extractor fans should be fitted into an outside wall, at high level, away from the door and near the cooker — it is best to seek expert advice on this from a local NICEIC (National Inspection Council for Electrical Installation and Contracting) electrical contractor (a list of contractors is kept by electricity shops and every electricity board is a registered contractor). The switch and other controls should be within reach and easy to manipulate. Cooker hoods either extract steam and smells by a vent pipe to the outside or clean the air by passing it through a charcoal filter which has to be replaced regularly.

Equipment such as a clothes dryer usually needs to be directly vented to the exterior in order to avoid condensation.

Refuse Disposal

A wide choice of bins and bags is available. People in wheelchairs find it almost impossible to reach those placed in cupboards under sinks, but bins can be mounted on pull-out tracks adjacent to the sink. Freestanding or wall-fixed bins with replaceable liners are convenient to use and to empty.

It is important that there should be easy access to a dustbin; it is sometimes possible to have a hatch, which must be well designed, from the kitchen to an external collection point.

Waste disposal units are usually sited under the sink which is inconvenient for wheelchair users; however, these units can be installed in other positions (such as in a corner) although this can be expensive unless the kitchen is being planned from scratch.

Safety (and Security)

Many points about safety in the kitchen (for instance, trailing flexes, slip-resistant floors and good lighting) have already been mentioned, or will be in the following chapters, and many are just good common sense (like avoiding clutter, wiping up spills and getting things repaired).

It is a good idea to have a small, safe fire extinguisher in an easily accessible place in the kitchen. Fire blankets, to smother a fire on the cooker, should be kept in the kitchen as a matter of course (Figure 1.13). DIY smoke detectors are available from many shops.

Rather than a fixed alarm bell, which may be out of reach, some people may prefer to carry one of the newer portable call systems, for example, a small alarm programmed to ring three telephone numbers to try and ensure that someone will answer (Figure 1.14).

Figure 1.13: Fire Blanket

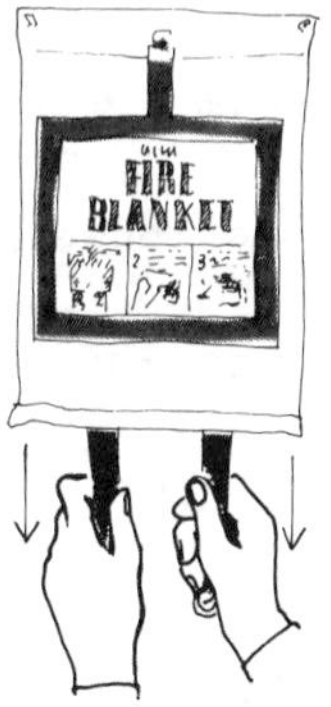

Figure 1.14: Portable Alarm Call System

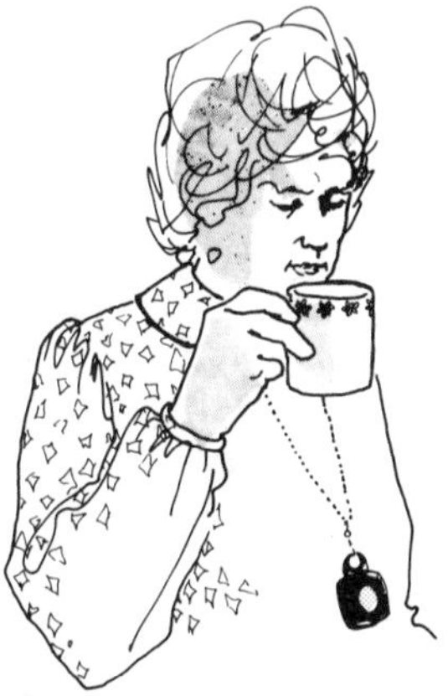

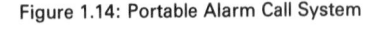

Many disabled and elderly people live on the ground floor or in bungalows and should be aware of the helpful advice which is available from the local police. Having stressed the importance of being able to open the kitchen window, it is equally important to remember to shut it at night and when you go out.

References

BS 5619 (1978) *Code of Practice for Design of Housing for the Convenience of Disabled People*
BS 6222: Part 1 (1982) *Domestic Kitchen Equipment Specification for Co-ordinating Dimensions*
Department of the Environment (1978) Circular 59/78, *Adaptations of Housing for People Who Are Physically Handicapped*
Electricity Council (1985) *Planning your Electric Kitchen*, EC (free)
Howie, P.M. (1967) *A Pilot Study of Disabled Housewives in their Kitchens*, Disabled Living Foundation
Goldsmith, S. (1974) 'Mobility housing', *Architects Journal*, July (reprinted as HDD Occasional Paper 2/74, Department of the Environment
— (1975) 'Wheelchair housing', *Architects Journal*, *25*, June (reprinted as HDD Occasional Paper 2/75, Department of the Environment)
— (1984) *Designing for the Disabled* (3rd edn, revised), RIBA Publications
Hillingdon, London Borough of (1980) *Clients' Opinions of Wheelchair Housing*, LBH
London Borough of (1980) *Clients' Opinions of Wheelchair Housing*, LBH
Institute of Housing/Royal Institute of British Architects (1983) *Homes for the Future*, IH/RIBA

2 Equipment

Gwen Conacher

There are two or three major items of equipment without which a kitchen cannot be a real workroom. Indeed, as shown in Chapter 1, they are integral parts of a good working kitchen and must be planned into the correct work sequence. These appliances are a cooker, refrigerator or fridge-freezer, a washing machine plus suitable drying facilities and, increasingly, a dishwasher. Although, ideally, the last three should be housed in a utility room, most people have to accommodate as much useful equipment as possible in a relatively small kitchen. If this space also has to allow for manoeuvring a wheelchair, even more careful consideration must be given to the choice of appliances and their placing; this is discussed in Chapter 1. No two people like exactly the same appliance or layout, and a kitchen must, above all else, be personal. If it cannot be perfect, it can be a happy, cheerful place; it will not work if the user has a lively hate of anything in it.

Fortunately, since essential appliances are available in a wide range of sizes and prices, it should be possible for everyone to find something to suit their needs. The best allies are the trained staff in the gas, solid fuel and electrical industries who will be happy to advise not only on the new models available, but also on some adapted controls for them, as well as for some existing appliances, if they are less than five years old. An increasing number of major appliances are being fitted with electronic controls which are bound to help people with disabilities.

Full-size Cookers

The cooker is the focal point of every kitchen. People make friends with their cookers and, for this reason, anyone who is suddenly afflicted with impaired vision, for instance, should be advised not to change the cooker immediately, because it is reassuring and easier to use a familiar appliance. You will find your hand goes to the right control almost by instinct. Similarly, if you face an increasing loss of strength or movement, it might be better to take time over choosing a more suitable appliance, until you have become acclimatised to personal limitations. The interim period can be used to assess what is available on the market.

When first faced with disablement, the temptation may be to make a clean sweep and change everything in the kitchen at once. Very often a change of layout works wonders, leaving tried and trusted friends like the cooker to be replaced when the time is right. If the controls on an existing cooker are increasingly difficult to use, it may well be possible to get alternative controls (see p. 26).

But when the time does come for a change, what is the choice, and what should you look for? The main choice is between gas and electric cookers, while modern solid fuel cookers are an alternative, especially in northern counties and country districts. This is a fundamental and very personal choice, and it is probably advisable to stick to the medium you are used to, unless you really want to change for reasons of cost, convenience, design or ease of use.

Generally speaking, both gas and electric cookers offer the basics — cooking hob with up to four individual rings, one oven, a grill and some means of heating serving dishes. Solid fuel cookers have more oven space, usually no grill and a large heated hob. The following sections detail the respective features of gas, electric and calor gas cookers. Choice starts with a basic cooker in a moderate price range and widens to include various other desirable, even essential, features in the higher price brackets. Descriptions of these additional features are given, the actual model specifications being available from the relevant retailing outlets.

If you are considering buying a new cooker, then read these sections carefully and ask to see one or two of the types that appeal to you most at the local shops. If you are unable to go yourself, get a relative or friend who knows your needs to assess them for you, or ask if a qualified adviser can visit you.

Finally, consider carefully whether a conventional floor-standing cooker is now the best choice. Would a split-level cooker be best so the cook-top and oven could each be placed at the best working height? Although this arrangement uses some extra working surface, remember that it makes more storage space and knee-room. Or, indeed, would a cooking hob alone be enough if you do not use the oven much? Perhaps an entirely different train of thought might indicate that a microwave cooker could solve a lot of problems or that several lighter, small, specialised cooking appliances might be easier and more versatile. All these alternatives are discussed. If you decide to keep to a standard cooker, consider getting a sturdy trolley to use with it, with shelf heights matching those of the oven and possibly the hob.

Gas Cookers

Each region of British Gas has a team of home service advisers who are happy to call on people at home to give free advice on any queries about choosing or using gas appliances. They give information and reassurance on the economical and safe use of gas, the importance of regular servicing and methods of payment. They also give helpful advice on choosing new appliances, from cookers to heating systems.

All home service advisers are in close contact with local authorities and social services departments and can therefore be of particular help to elderly and disabled people — especially where help is needed with special aids for appliances. Contact the local home service adviser either through your local British Gas showroom or service centre which is listed under 'Gas' in the telephone directory.

Types and Sizes of Gas Cookers. When buying a new cooker, it is better to go to a British Gas showroom or authorised dealer, as these are backed by the full after-sales services of British Gas. Gas cookers are made in a number of different styles to suit a variety of needs, but most are designed to fit into, or line up with, standard kitchen units.

1. Free-standing. These cookers consist of a grill, hotplate and oven placed one above the other to form one unit. On some cookers, the grill is placed between the hotplate and oven at a low level, and on others it is above the hotplate at high level. Free-standing cookers are usually between 457 mm (18 in) and 610 mm (24 in) wide and the hotplate between 864 mm (34 in) and 914 mm (36 in) from the floor. For a cooker with a high level grill, a clear space of at least 457 mm (18 in) must be left above and 100 mm (4 in) either side of the grill.

Some models can be fitted between kitchen units to give a 'built-in' appearance. These particular flush-fitting cookers usually have a fold-down lid, and are referred to as 'slide-in' appliances.

2. Range. These cookers usually have two ovens side by side with a high or low level grill, and are usually more than 635 mm (25 in) wide.

3. Table-top. This is a smaller version of a free-standing cooker with two burners, a small oven and a grill. This compact cooker can be obtained on a stand or as separate units.

4. Built-in. The oven, hotplate and grill are bought as separate units so that they can be built into kitchen units at a convenient height to suit the individual. They come in a number of variations such as combined oven/grills, double oven/grills, units incorporating a microwave oven and built-under units. Built-in units are usually the most suitable for people in wheelchairs or those who find it difficult to reach up or down as they can be fitted at any convenient height into most makes of kitchen furniture (Figure 2.1). It is also possible to buy special kitchen units designed for disabled users into which these cookers will fit.

The Grill

Many free-standing gas cooker grills are at high level, although some low level grills are becoming more popular. It should be remembered that in the latter case the oven will be lower down and the drawer omitted. Some grills have a fixed compartment for the grill pan to fit into and others can be folded away when not in use. Most grills have at least two grilling positions

Figure 2.1: Built-in Gas Cooker

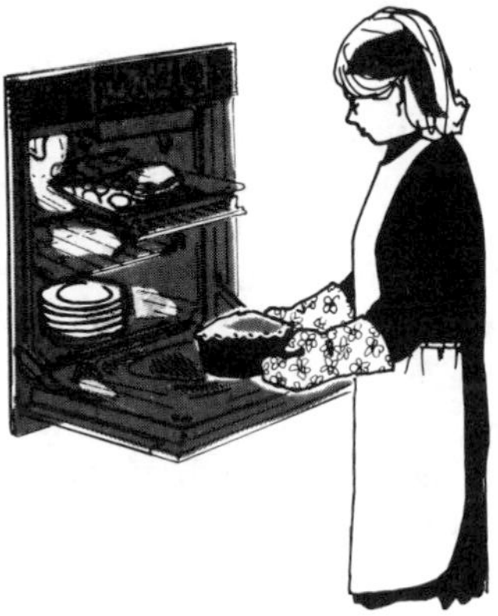

with room for warming plates, and the grill pans have either one or two handles.

The grill pan will either sit on a shelf, slide in on a runner, or can sometimes be fixed to a device which allows the pan to be drawn forward and held in position safely so that food can be turned over. The heat is adjusted by turning the flame up or down as required. A surface combustion grill gives an even heat over the whole area at every heat setting. Rotisseries and duplex burners are available as optional extras on some grills.

The Hob

This usually has four burners which can be of different sizes — large ones for fast cooking and smaller ones for simmering — but generally they are all the same size because they are all quick and easy to control. On most cookers the burners are set into a sealed hotplate top which makes cleaning much easier. Pan supports can be either individual over each burner, over two burners or cover the whole hotplate top. Modern burners are easy to light either by a piezo spark, a battery spark or mains electric spark, none of which requires much pressure. These operate automatically as the burner control is turned on or by pushing a button. Batteries operate the piezo ignition, but remember that an electric ignition system must have an electric socket outlet near the cooker. Some ignition systems have a re-ignition device as a special safety feature which automatically relights the burner if it goes out accidentally. Other special features on a hotplate are thermostatically controlled burners, simmer–stop positions on burners, visual indicators to show when burners are lit, griddle plates and fold-down lids.

The Oven

Heat in the oven of a British gas cooker is zoned, as the burner is usually situated in the base at the back of the oven and heat circulates up and around the oven space. This means that dishes which require different temperatures can be cooked together and the whole of the oven used, which is a good way of saving energy. There is no need to pre-heat the oven as the heat is instant — the only exception is for dishes which require a very critical temperature such as soufflés. All standard sized cookers are fitted with a thermostat to control the temperature, and some have a special slow setting. The number on the control when set refers to the temperature in the middle of the oven. There can be four to seven shelf positions in the oven, always counted from the top downwards and two shelves are provided with each cooker.

To make cleaning easier, cookers are usually fitted with linings that help to keep themselves clean. These work continuously and just need an occasional wipe over. Ovens have drop-down doors or side-opening doors that can be hinged either left or right, whichever is the most convenient. These can have a glass panel in them with a light in the oven, so you can see exactly what is happening to the cooking. Ignition again is by either piezo, battery or electric spark, and all cookers have flame failure devices — a special safety feature that ensures no gas will come through to the oven burner should it go out for any reason.

Several other special features on gas ovens include automatic cooking controls, clocks, minute minders, rotisseries and kebab attachments.

Special Controls

Most controls on gas cookers are conveniently situated on the front fascia panel. For those with hand disabilities, British Gas has developed a range of specially designed controls for cookers. Four types of tap handle — designed in conjunction with specialist organisations to suit the needs of various disabilities — are available for a wide range of cookers, including some older models (Figure 2.2). Tap B, for example, has been found to be most suitable for someone with weakness in the arm due to polio or muscular dystrophy. A small nominal charge is made for these handles, details of

Figure 2.2: Special Controls for Gas Cookers: (a) Large, Lumpy Handle which is Easy to Grip, Especially for Arthritis Sufferers; (b) Lever to Help People with General Weakness of the Arm and Hand; (c) People with Poor Muscular Co-ordination or Tremor Should Find the Projections on this Handle Easier to Grip; (d) Tap Handle with Detachable Lever Especially Suited to Cookers with Controls Set Close Together; (e) Special Braille or Studded Oven Thermostat Dial

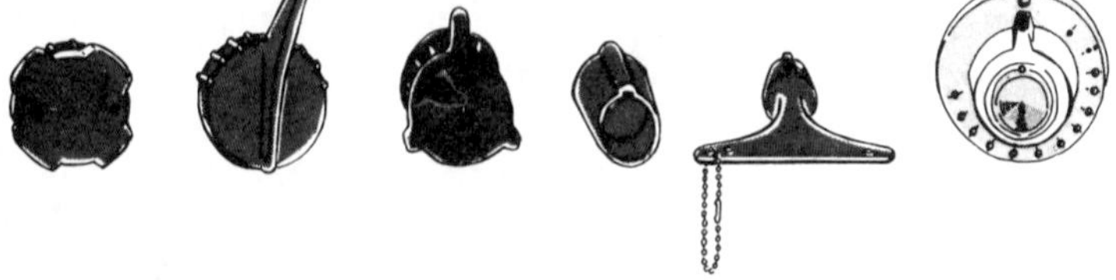

which are given in a leaflet *Advice for Disabled People* (see Appendix III, p. 157). Adaptors are also available for most fires and wall-heaters.

For users with a visual impairment, it is possible to get braille or studded controls (Figure 2.2e), together with a braille cooking chart, to make cooking a little easier. Some gas regions also have recipe tapes which are helpful to blind people; ask the home service adviser for details. A pre-payment gas meter fitted in an awkward position which makes it impossible to manage can be repositioned at a more convenient height at a specially reduced cost. (When meters are replaced as part of British Gas meter replacement programme, they are usually sited externally where practicable, and no charge is made.) In addition, a special extension can be fitted to make the meter handle easier to turn. Details of all these special services may be obtained from the local home service adviser.

LPG Cookers

Those who prefer a gas cooker but do not have access to mains gas, have a wide range of models available for use with liquefied petroleum gas (LPG). Calor is the leading UK supplier of LPG and appliances are available from Calor dealers and Calor centres (addresses in British Telecom's *Yellow Pages* under 'Bottled Gas'). These cookers can be operated from either a cylinder installation or a bulk tank, depending on requirements and whether central heating by Calor Gas is also required.

LPG cookers, although visually identical to their mains gas counterparts, do have technical differences, so units designed for LPG use must never be interchanged with those designed for mains gas use.

Features of these cookers, which are available either as free-standing or built-in versions, include timers, rotisseries, push-button ignition and self-cleaning ovens. Supply of gas is trouble-free, as bulk tanks are replenished by road delivery vehicles and cylinders can be replaced by the local stockist.

Electric Cookers

Most electric cookers have similar dimensions to standard kitchen floor-standing furniture units (that is, approximately 600 mm (24 in) square and 900 mm (36 in) high). This makes it easy to move pans to either side of the cooker by sliding them across onto the recommended adjacent working surface (Figure 2.3a). They usually have vitreous enamel hobs, in which are set three or four radiant boiling rings. The oven is at the bottom of the cooker and the grill is usually under the hob, set in a shallower compartment which also acts as a plate warming area and very often as a complete second oven. At least one has the grill and second oven placed at the back of the cooker at high level. The switches on the front of this grill and on some small table-top ovens (Figure 2.3b) are particularly useful to people with poor sight.

Figure 2.3a: Floor-standing Electric Cooker

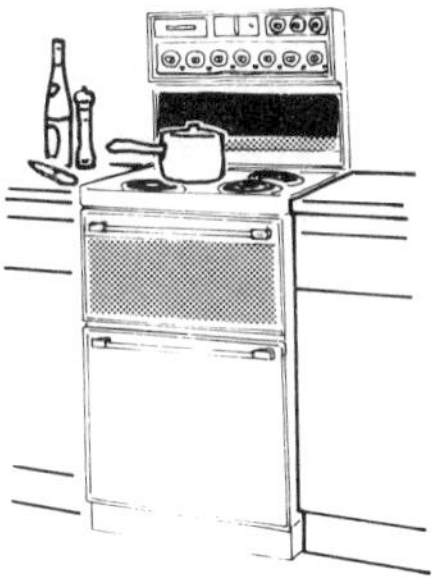

Figure 2.3b: Table-top Oven with Boiling Rings

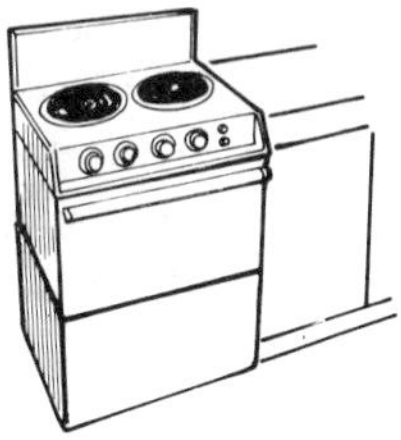

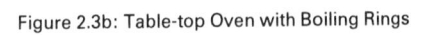

The Cooking Hob

This is usually indented to catch any spills and is easily wiped clean with a damp cloth. Most also have spillage trays underneath the rings which can be removed and taken to the sink for cleaning. Those with single dishes, or half-width trays, are easiest to handle.

The radiant rings glow red at the highest setting, but for the best and most economical cooking results, they should always be set at the lowest suitable setting for the cooking job being done. This saves splashes too. Most cookers, except the very basic ones, have at least one 'dual-control' ring; this means that either the whole or the small central element can be used. The small ring is very useful for small pans and for gentle simmering.

Ceramic hobs are a fairly recent development in cooker design (Figure 2.3c). They may be part of a standard cooker or can be set into a work surface at any convenient height, like conventional separate hobs, which is advantageous for a chairbound user. They consist of a smooth sheet of tough, heat-resistant brown or black glass over four separate elements, the position of which is marked on the glass. They are easy to keep clean if the instructions are followed and the prescribed cleaning products are used. However, if you cannot lift heavy pans and prefer to slide them, it is as well to know that this continual sliding could cause scratch marks which are impossible to remove.

Figure 2.3c: Ceramic Hob

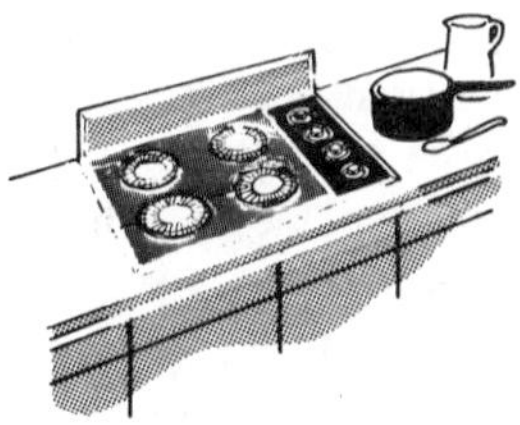

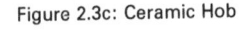

Full details of these hobs are given on an information sheet available from Electricity Boards. A device on some of the elements of the latest ceramic hob brings the pan very quickly to the desired boiling or simmering level and holds it there with electronic precision. A new version of these hobs incorporates cooking areas heated by 'halogen heat'. This comes from tungsten/halogen lamps which give a very bright light; this decreases in strength as the heat is lowered so that it is possible to 'see' the heat level.

The Grill

This is heated by one or two radiant elements. Some have a separate control for half the cooking area (either one side, or the central area only) which is useful when grilling small quantities of food for one or two people.

The grill pan and/or its cradle or shelf can be pulled out to a workable distance, thanks to a variety of safe non-tip devices. Grill pans can have one or two handles according to the model — make sure to choose one which you can manage comfortably.

The grill chamber is used also for warming dishes, and on a number of models can also be used as a completely separate fully heated and auto-timed oven.

The door of the grill compartment opens downwards on strong hinges, so that it can be used as a serving shelf.

The Oven

All the oven space in an electric cooker is usable, so that it is quite big enough for the normal family requirements as well as for just one dish. Even so, as with all other types of cookers, if you are energy-conscious, it is advisable to plan oven cooking so that it is not used too often for single items.

The heat is even and steady throughout the oven, and there is no need to pre-heat the oven except for food needing a high temperature for a short time, such as a Swiss roll.

Some cookers incorporate a fan oven. Not only are these even more economical, but they contain up to four shelves, all of which can be packed and used together. Such cookers are ideal for those who like baking because, on a 'good' day, a stock of cakes and pastry can be baked and stored in the freezer. Oven doors are usually hinged on the left, but some can be simply reversed; quite a few of them also have inner glass doors, which could be a mixed blessing for one-handed people.

Most electric ovens now have 'stay-clean' surfaces which eliminate the difficult job of cleaning and it is well worth choosing one with this surface treatment should a conventionally heated oven be the choice.

Controls

Cooker controls are simple variations on knobs which turn. The oven control incorporates a thermostat, and most cookers have an additional auto-timing oven control. Although manufacturers continue to improve the design and placing of cooker controls, bearing in mind ergonomic factors, it is difficult for people with some disablements of the hands or arms to reach or use them easily. Consequently, all major British manufacturers have made available sets of alternative controls which are free of charge to disabled people. Ask about them at your Electricity Board shop when ordering a new cooker. In some cases, it may be possible to fit them to an existing cooker at a nominal charge — ask your Board about this, too.

People with sight defects should enquire about good colour contrast between the switches and their background, and about the special tactile features on most cooker controls. Electricity Boards are always pleased to help with specialised problems. Most of them offer a special 'identification' method of introducing any employee who has to call at the home of a sight-impaired customer.

Built-in or 'Split-level' Cooker

Several versions of the popular divided cooker are now available. The oven/grill units are designed to fit into a properly built casing supplied by most leading kitchen unit manufacturers, including those offering special ranges for disabled people. One supplier also makes a very small free-standing cooker with two rings, available as well in two parts — oven/grill and hob (Figure 2.3b).

A wide variety of separate 'drop-in' hobs lends versatility to this type of cooker. They are particularly useful for people working from wheelchairs, because they can be set at any convenient height, with the switches to the left, right or front of the rings, wherever they are easiest to reach. The oven/grill units may have the grill above or below the oven and the main oven doors can be hinged on either right or left. The controls are usually on the front, above the doors. If at all possible, try handling a unit in a shop where one is displayed before buying.

Continental Cookers

Recently, a number of imported electric and gas cookers of European design have appeared on the British market. At first sight, they seem to incorporate many features suitable for disabled people. Generally smaller than British cookers, they are also shallower, because the grill is in the oven and there is no separate grill chamber; and they have the switches at the front.

However, it is important to remember that they were designed for continental cooks and are not designed primarily to cook a good Victoria sandwich, fruit cake or roast joint — three favourite British standbys — which are all in the British Standard for cookers, to which all British cookers are made. Many purchasers have discovered this to their cost, plus the fact that the boiling discs, being less powerful than British ones, are much slower. It is fair to say that most continental manufacturers are working on this problem and have employed British home economists to compile instructions and recipe books for British food cooked in their cookers. British cooker manufacturers, too, are now offering alternative models which combine the best of continental design with the ability to cook food to British Standard requirements (Figure 2.3d).

Cleaning the Cooker

The cooker itself can be wiped clean easily and, if you choose an oven with 'stay-clean' surface, you will be free of the worst of oven cleaning chores. The vitreous enamel hob is easy to wipe clean when still warm. Obstinate stains can be loosened by wetting them well or by using an all-purpose cleansing liquid. Visually handicapped people can often feel grease and food deposits and, when cleaning the cooker top, should use the same methodical routine each time so that the whole surface is covered. However, the glass door and shelves may need cleaning from time to time and the following tested tips may help you. For those who have not got an oven with a stay-clean finish, pointers on cleaning vitreous enamel ovens are also included.

1. Do not let grease splashes build up and burn on. Try to wipe round the oven after each use. This is unnecessary with stay-clean sides, but the shelves and doors should have regular attention.
2. If the shelves, sides and base of the oven, and the spill trays from under the rings are removable, take them to the sink where it is easier to tackle them.
3. Soak removable parts (without a stay-clean finish) in a strong hot detergent or soda solution, which will loosen the dirt, making it easier to wash off with an abrasive pad. Special biological washing powders in solution also loosen stains very well.
4. Proprietary oven cleaners may be used, providing the manufacturers' instructions can be carefully followed. Do not use them on stay-clean surfaces, or attempt to scrub these surfaces in any way. They should always

Figure 2.3d: Slip-in Freestanding Electric Cooker

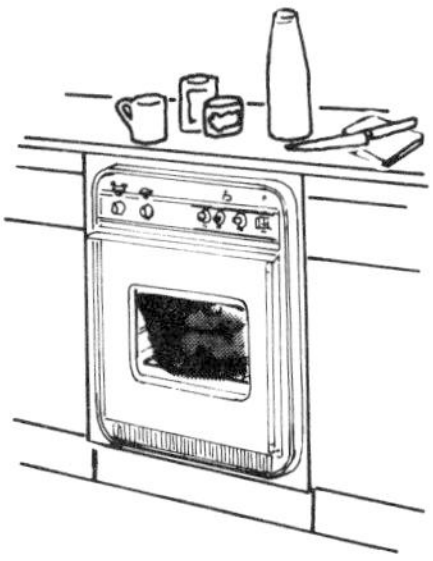

stay presentably clean, but any thick splashes can be removed by washing in hot water and detergent.

5. Use the food trolley, covered with newspaper, to hold the removable pieces until returned.

6. If you have any kind of skin trouble, whether the hands are affected or not, it is wise to wear rubber gloves (preferably with cotton or silk linings) while using strong detergent, soda, proprietary oven cleaners or biological powders. Make sure these protective gloves come well up the arms (see also the section on oven gloves in Chapter 3).

7. For those suffering from respiratory diseases (asthma, bronchitis, recurrent pneumonia or any other lung or bronchial disease), 'spray on' oven cleaners are best avoided unless extreme care is taken to avoid accidental inhalation of the sprayed material. A warm, damp face mask is best, but a clean damp teacloth makes a good substitute.

Safety and Service

Electricity

All British electric cookers are made to conform with the requirements of BS 3456 (1969) *Specification for Safety of Household and Similar Appliances* and carry the BEAB label of the British Electrotechnical Approvals Board (Figure 2.4). This means that they have been type-tested and approved for electrical safety in accordance with British Standards.

Modifications or repairs to cookers should never be attempted by an unqualified person. Always ask the Electricity Board or other qualified electrician to do electrical work. Names and addresses of electrical contractors recognised by the NICEIC (National Inspection Council for Electrical Installation and Contracting) can be obtained through the Electricity Boards. Their telephone numbers are shown in local directories under 'Electricity'.

Figure 2.4: BEAB Labels: from 1986 (a) will be gradually phased out in favour of (b) and (c)

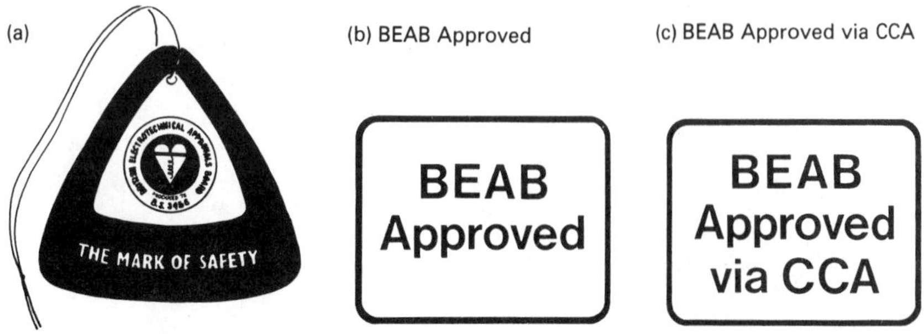

Be very wary about buying a secondhand cooker or any other secondhand electrical appliance. Buy only from an accredited supplier (see previous paragraph) and make sure that the cooker carries BEAB approval and that spares are available for that particular model. Although secondhand appliances may be cheaper to buy initially, they may not last long or perform efficiently, so that they may turn out to be more expensive in the long run. Again, never let a 'handyman' install an electric cooker for you. Make sure it is installed by the Electricity Board or other qualified electrician. They can usually be fixed quite easily with correct wiring and a control panel, wherever in the kitchen is most convenient, but preferably not in front of a window.

Gas

Safety and service are a major priority to British Gas. Gas is a safe fuel, but like any source of energy should always be treated with respect. British Gas and all appliance manufacturers work hard to make sure that all appliances are safe to use.

Most appliances sold by British Gas have been certified for conformity to British Standards by the Certification and Assessment Service of the British Standards Institution. This is an independent body which monitors the testing and manufacture of new gas appliances against the requirements of British Standards. Before they receive a licence to use the 'Safety Mark' manufacturers must satisfy the relevant safety standards. In the case of the 'Kitemark' the standards cover not only safety but performance as well (Figure 2.5a). Appliances not covered by the BSI scheme are tested by British Gas to the relevant British Standard.

Every gas appliance sold and installed by British Gas is also covered by the 'Seal of Service' for one year (Figure 2.5b). This is a comprehensive guarantee covering the appliance, its installation, the availability of spare parts and the workmanship of the British Gas staff who install and service it.

Once you have bought a gas appliance, it is important to make sure that

Figure 2.5a: BSI 'Safety Mark' and 'Kitemark'

Figure 2.5b: British Gas 'Seal of Service'

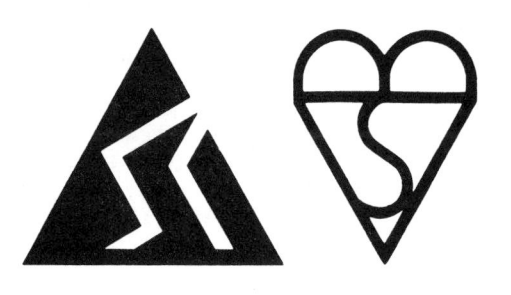

any service to it is carried out by a British Gas service engineer or a CORGI registered installer; never rely on an unqualified person. Gas fires, boilers and water heaters need checking once a year. There are a number of contract servicing schemes available to arrange this.

You may be entitled to a free gas safety check if you are a registered disabled person of any age and live alone, or if you are over 65 and live alone. This check includes any necessary adjustments and materials up to an agreed limit of value. If the check shows that more costly repairs should be made, you can be given an official estimate. The local social services department or Social Security office may be able to help meet the cost, but remember to ask before ordering any work to be done. Contact your local British Gas Showroom or Service Centre to arrange for this check, or other work.

All British Gas employees who have reason to call on customers carry an identity card. Ask to see this before admitting anyone. Calls are rarely made unexpectedly — except in the case of the meter reader. It is for this reason that a 'password' scheme operates for blind customers (Figure 2.6a). The password, chosen by the customer, is known only by the British Gas Region concerned and is quoted by the meter reader to enable the blind person to check his/her identity.

Gas Leaks. If you smell gas: (1) put out cigarettes; do not use matches or naked flames; (2) do not operate electrical switches on or off (including doorbells); (3) if you are able, open doors and windows to get rid of the gas; (4) turn off at the meter and call Gas Service, listed under 'Gas' in telephone directory (Figure 2.6b).

Checking a suspected leak will usually be free of charge because the first 30 minutes of work is not charged for, including small value parts and materials.

If you find your main gas tap is stiff and will not turn properly, do not force it. Ask your local gas service centre to loosen it free of charge.

Practical Safety Measures

If you suffer from any kind of skin condition, even though the face and hands are not affected, consider carefully before deciding upon the type of oven door to be bought. Heat 'blast' from a hot oven can damage susceptible skins. Heat blast travels sideways from a side-opening door and upwards from a door hinged at the bottom. Be sure that there is ample room at the side of, or in front of, the oven door to avoid the risk of a rush of hot air. It is not always so noticeable with some makes of fan-assisted ovens.

Do not dry tea-towels by hanging them above or on the cooker.

Figure 2.6a: British Gas 'Password' Scheme

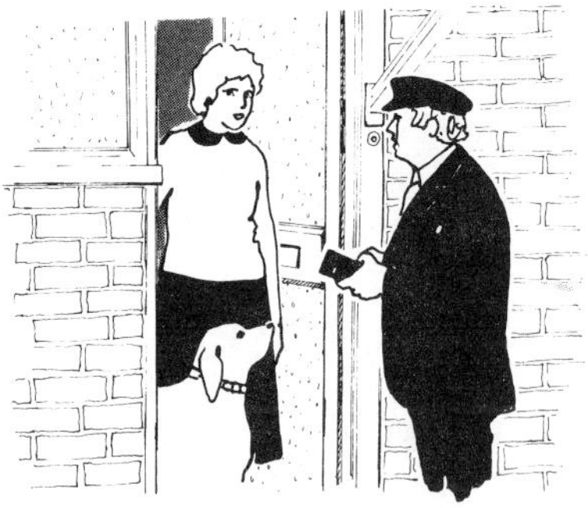

Figure 2.6b: Gas Meter Handle Showing 'Off' and 'On' Positions

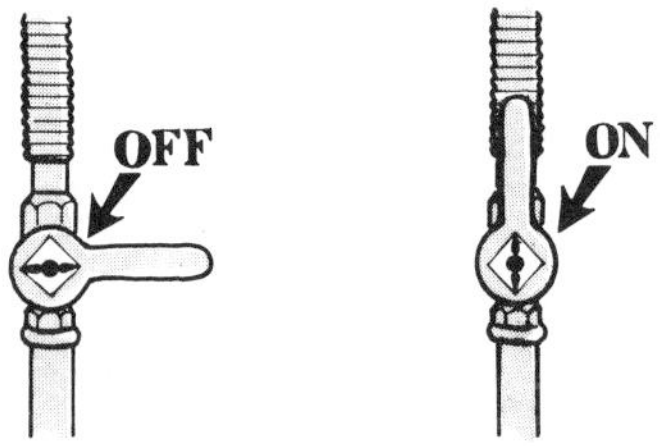

Keep all saucepan handles turned away from the front edge of the cooker.

Use oven gloves, preferably long ones which cover the forearms.

Finally, do not let electrical flexes from kettles or other appliances lie across the cooker.

Running Costs

Contrary to popular belief, cooking is *not* an extravagant use of energy. Plenty of information about wise ways of using and conserving heat and energy is available from the appropriate authorities, but here it is probably sufficient to indicate that the cost of electricity and gas for cooking is just a small fraction of the cost of the ingredients, or even of one ingredient of any one dish.

Oven Temperature Equivalents

Since 1975, electric ovens have been calibrated in the metric system, using degrees Celsius (°C). The following chart gives both the original Fahrenheit scale and the present Celsius scale, compared with the gas oven marks. Most cookery writers and editors use the three equivalent settings in their recipes, but this chart will help you to use old favourite recipes with a new cooker.

Gas mark	*Electric* °F	*Electric* °C
1/4	225	110
1/2	250	120
1	275	140
2	300	150
3	325	160

Gas mark	*Electric* °F	*Electric* °C
4	350	180
5	375	190
6	400	200
7	425	220
8	450	230
9	475	240

Choosing a Cooker

Before making a final choice of a new cooker, use this check list.

1. Can you reach the grill? If it is a high-level one, has it got a stop to prevent the pan falling out when pulled forward?
2. Can you manage the control knobs safely and easily or will you require alternative knobs? If the oven you are considering is a gas model, it is likely that the knob will need to be pushed and turned.
3. Can you manage the oven shelves? Ideally, you should be able to pull them out part way without them coming out completely.
4. Would a drop-down or side-opening door suit you better? A drop-down door can be used as a shelf for dishes before lifting them up, but may present difficulties to a wheelchair user. If a side-opening door, should it open to left or right? Can you open the door easily?
5. Is the hob stable for pans?
6. Will cleaning the cooker be a problem? Will the top need taking apart to clean and has the oven got a stay-clean lining?
7. Do you need plate-warming facilities?
8. Would an automatic oven which can be pre-set to switch on and off at a set time help you? Could you operate this timer or would someone else do this for you?

In addition, a visually handicapped person should remember:

1. to look for good contrast between the markings on the knobs and the background panel. Alternatively, the knobs can be marked with Hi-Marks (see p. 62);
2. that sealed hot plates, a lift-up top and individual spillage bowls make cleaning easier (but see point 5 below);
3. that the controls must be positioned so that there is no risk of leaning across the burners to reach them;
4. that spark ignition is safer than matches;
5. that continuous pan supports minimise the risk of toppling (although they may be less easy to clean, see point 2 above);
6. that knobs with a raised bar across are ideal for regulating using the 'clock' method;

7. the advantages of having an eye-level grill with stops and a two-handled pan with front and rear stops.

Ask at the local gas or electricity showroom about the availability of adapted knobs for the particular model chosen.

Table Top Cookers

As already mentioned, a considerable range of efficient small electric cooking appliances is on the market. These offer quick and economical results and, because of their portability and general versatility, some of them are especially useful to disabled people.

All these appliances (discussed on the following pages) do what their manufacturers claim for them, but you will not want all of them. Choose from those which best fit your lifestyle, either because they specialise in cooking the food you like to eat, or because they can be tackled more easily than a conventional cooker, or both. All can be used on any work surface, connected to a 13 amp socket outlet, and should be kept easily to hand. To help you to choose, brief comments are included about each range and detailed information and specification sheets on all these appliances are obtainable from the manufacturers or from Electricity Boards. Always choose only those models which carry BEAB approval.

Contact Grills

Sometimes known as infra-red grills, these consist of two electrically heated plates, hinged together (Figure 2.7). The plates have a non-stick coating and the upper plate is self-adjusting to accommodate different thicknesses of food or a shallow cooking tray. All food which is normally grilled, and most which is normally fried, can be cooked in a contact grill, with little or no extra fat. The tray can be used to cook small quantities of simple cakes

Figure 2.7: Contact Grill

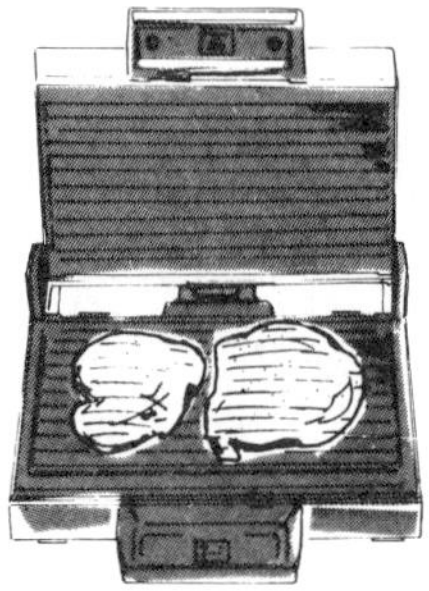

Figure 2.8: Sandwich Toaster

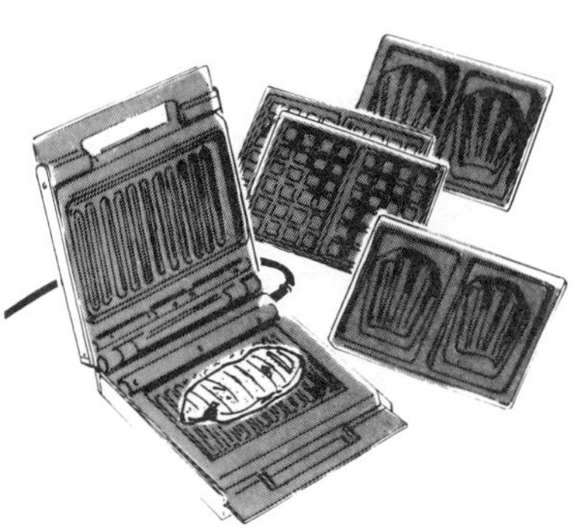

and pastry, or for rapid thawing and cooking of frozen food. For ease of cleaning, choose those with removable plates.

Sandwich Toasters

Sandwiches can be toasted in a contact grill, but a specialised sandwich toaster does an even better job, because it has shaped hollows to take more sandwich filling, sealing the edges so that the contents cannot escape (Figure 2.8). Although more limited in application than the contact grill, it is smaller and lighter and a surprising variety of really nutritious light snacks, both savoury and sweet, can be made in it. Some of the larger ones may be rather heavy to lift open.

Toasters

Toasters were among the first electric appliances and have proved their worth (Figure 2.9). More economical to use than a large cooker grill, they push the bread up automatically when toasted so that there is no need to watch the bread cooking. Modern versions include slide controls to give choice of brownness, some adjusting themselves electronically to the freshness or otherwise of the bread. Most have two really wide slots to take muffins or crumpets and some toast four slices of bread at once. Some control levers move more easily than others.

Toaster Ovens

A few appliances combine the functions of the previous three. Toaster ovens are really very small ovens which can take two slices of bread, a small tray of buns or a couple of chops, grill bacon and sausages, or toast a sandwich (Figure 2.10). One also has slots for toasting bread like a conventional toaster. For a single person they offer versatile cooking for a wide range of food, especially for anyone prepared to experiment. Some are a little awkward to clean.

Figure 2.9: Toaster

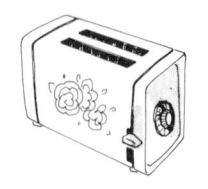

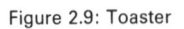

Figure 2.10: Toaster Oven

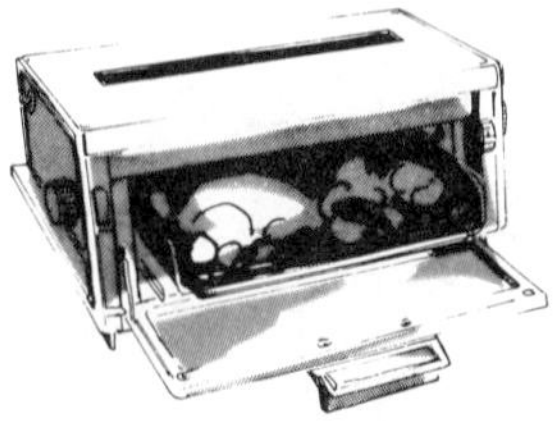

Multi-purpose Cookers

These are well named. Originally known as electric frying pans, these appliances now have a variety of applications and make excellent complete cookers for one or two people (Figure 2.11). They can be square or round and have a domed lid, and can be used for frying, boiling, stewing, roasting and even baking. The control/thermostat with indicator light can be unplugged from the cooker and as the heating element is completely enclosed, the whole pan can be washed. But most have a non-stick interior coating, so cleaning is easy. Some are heavier than others. Try for ease of lifting before buying.

Deep-fat Fryers

This more specialised appliance makes an important contribution to kitchen safety. It is designed primarily for deep frying, heating the oil thermostatically to the correct safe temperature (Figure 2.12). Since it cannot overheat there is no danger of the oil self-igniting and, because this is one form of deep frying where a lid can be used, splashing and bubbling over are prevented. Some models have a filter in the lid to prevent greasy steam permeating the kitchen. A frying basket is supplied which can usually be raised and lowered without opening the lid.

As the oil does not overheat, it can be cooled and stored in the container, but does need straining and changing occasionally. This is an awkward job to carry out unassisted, but there are a few small fryers for one or two people which are easier to lift. If required, the big fryers can be used for jobs like blanching vegetables before freezing but, as this entails draining and cleaning the pan, it may not be easy for everyone.

Slow-cooking Pots

At the other end of the scale from all the fast cookers, is a range of earthenware cooking pots with very low electric loadings, designed to cook food very slowly indeed, requiring no attention at all (Figure 2.13). For this reason, they are ideal for someone with severely restricted movement or

Figure 2.11: Multi-purpose Cooker

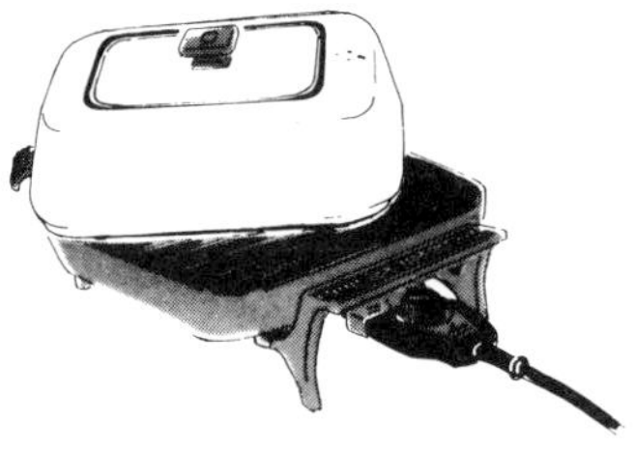

Figure 2.12: Deep-fat Fryer

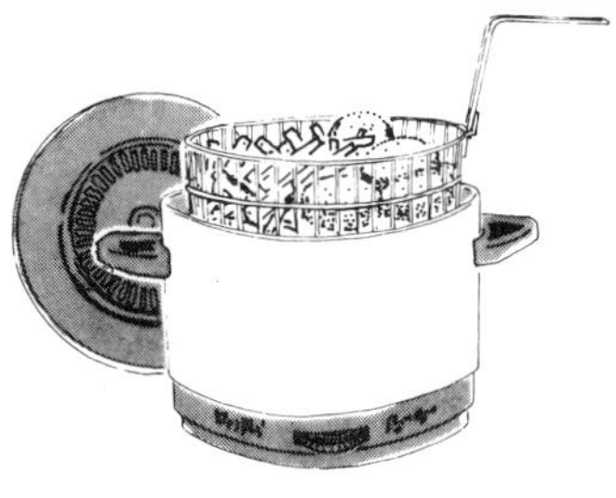

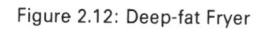

Figure 2.13: Slow-cooking Pot

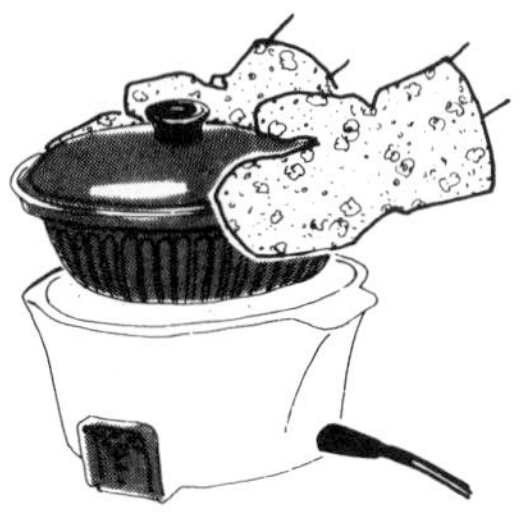

someone with poor vision, especially if a helper is able to start the cooking process, leaving the user to serve himself after several hours when the food is cooked. They are also good for someone who feels energetic early in the day, but who tires quickly. Stews, casseroles, soups and fruit all cook beautifully in a slow cooker, but these cookers also cope with steamed puddings and with cooking tongue and some preserves. Full instructions for use come with every model.

The very big family-size models usually have an additional automatic control to switch the cooker down once the food is heated though. The standard and smaller versions usually operate on one heat only. Although gentle and steady, the temperature is high enough to avoid any worry about bacterial contamination. After cooking, any remaining food should be transferred to another container and kept in the refrigerator in the usual way. Some have a removable inner container, but these may be difficult to lift. Smaller versions of these appliances are most easily lifted and handled by the majority of disabled people.

Although the cookers should not be immersed in water, they can be cleaned by standing them in the empty sink and rinsing them with hot water and a brush.

Microwave Cookers

Microwave cookers offer a totally different method of cooking which has many advantages, not least to the disabled cook, so it is well worth spending a little time on finding out about them if you are interested; and be prepared to find that new cooking techniques need to be mastered during the first few weeks of ownership.

What is meant by microwave cooking? A microwave cooker works by generating electromagnetic waves — the same sort of short, invisible, unfelt waves that bring us radio and television. The cooker itself is virtually a small box (or 'oven' as it is sometimes called) in which electricity is converted into these electromagnetic waves, and contains them within its metal lining (Figure 2.14). Microwaves cannot penetrate metal, so the waves are

Figure 2.14: Microwave Cooker

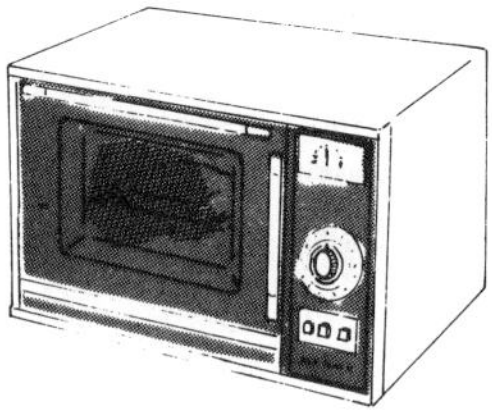

reflected across the cooking cavity from side to side and from top to bottom. They can penetrate other substances, which means that any material except metal can be used for cooking containers, and they are absorbed by moisture, contained in all food. As the microwaves are absorbed, they cause the moisture molecules in the food to vibrate, which causes heat and cooks the food. Although some foods take approximately the same time to cook as by conventional methods, others cook very much faster, so conserving energy and nutrients.

The following are the advantages of microwave cooking for the disabled user.

1. The cooker is comparatively small, can be set at any height on any sturdy work surface, in any suitable room and simply needs connecting to a standard electric socket outlet with a 13amp plug.
2. It is completely safe. Choose a model carrying BEAB approval (see p. 32) which means that it has been type tested to British Standards for electrical safety and microwave leakage. Approved models have many safety features, including a series of positive door locks, seals and switches, which make it impossible to operate the cooker without the door being tightly shut. Opening the door immediately stops microwave generation. There are no hot surfaces, inside or outside the cooker, so it is impossible to get a burn through accidentally touching the cooker — a point to be appreciated by people who have minimal sight. Some cooking dishes get hot, being heated by the food itself, so it is wise to use oven gloves when removing them.
3. The microwave cooker is easy to clean. As the sides of the cooker do not get hot, splashes do not bake on, and a light wipe with a clean damp cloth is all that is required. Most food can be covered to prevent spattering.
4. As all cooking is done inside the single cavity, no separate boiling rings are required. For the same reason, food can often be cooked in its serving dish (or drinks heated in a cup) so saving on utensils and washing up.
5. The controls are few and simple, usually consisting of a simple on/off button and a big easily turned dial for timing. The timer automatically

switches the cooker off at the set time.

6. The controls are reasonably tactile, but several manufacturers have alternative sets of brailled controls for people with impaired sight. In addition, the controls are all quite audible — there is a low hum during operation and a bell or pinger indicates when the cooker has switched off.

7. Lightweight dishes and containers can be used (an exception is some plastic, which warps with the high temperatures of hot fat or sugar) to make lifting easier. Very little water need be added to vegetables. Some foods can be cooked in plastic bags or covered with cling film, which means less washing up. Be careful to open bags and remove cling film away from you — using some protection from the steam.

8. Most food cooks in a fraction of the conventional time (steamed puddings in 10 minutes, for instance) and frozen food can be thawed very quickly in a microwave cooker.

9. The cooker is invaluable for reheating food on the plate for slow eaters.

Because microwave cooking is a moist method of cooking, food does not brown in the conventional way. The various ways of overcoming this are set out in the many cookery books now available on the subject. Cakes can be simply decorated, chops can be lightly grilled first, and joints and poultry can be dusted with one of the savoury browning preparations available.

Microwave Safety and Health. When doctors first started to fit patients with heart 'pacemakers', they warned them to keep away from microwave cookers. Nowadays, however, pacemakers fitted to patients in the UK are properly suppressed and completely unaffected by microwaves.

The National Radiological Protection Board has stated that it is 'not aware of any proven substantive cases where users of heart pacemakers have suffered serious ill-effects from microwave radiation, and would not expect these when wearers of modern pacemakers are not exposed above UK limits. This can reasonably be assumed for other implants such as metal plates and joints, but local field concentrations could arise within the body with consequential local heating.'

Small Appliances (Not Cookers) as Useful Adjuncts to Cooking

Many small electric domestic appliances, because they use a small electric motor, do a number of routine kitchen jobs quickly and well. They are useful to everyone; doubly so to those suffering some form of disablement. Others, with variations on the heating theme, are also invaluable both because they are quick and can be used exactly where required. Again, some will have more appeal than others to a particular individual, and the following list will serve as a reminder of what is available. All can be used from a 13amp socket outlet and BEAB-approved models should be chosen. A selection of each type of small appliance is usually available at most major electrical retail outlets: Electricity Board shops; electrical shops and stores; department stores. Although it is rarely possible to find every item available to try, it is sometimes possible to lift and handle display models. Large stores frequently stage practical demonstrations of manufacturers' branded appliances which help individual assessment. Fully detailed data sheets about each group of appliances are available (see p. 157).

Kettles

Some form of heating small quantities of water is essential in the kitchen, but the conventional kettle may not always be the best utensil (see p. 100 for non-electric kettles).

Electric kettles can be used in any room, and on most surfaces, as they have insulated feet (Figure 2.15). Although many are available with manual control (that is, the user must turn them off at the socket outlet when they boil), a great many are now automatic and turn themselves off when they come to the boil. It is well worth getting one of these although the initial outlay is higher. Not only are they more economical in use, but they do not fill a room with steam, and save the user from worrying about trying to hurry to switch them off. All models have a safety cut-out which turns the kettle off should it be turned on accidentally when empty.

Sometimes people living alone ask if there is a small electric kettle available. The few that are on the market cost nearly as much as the standard 1.7 litre (3 pint) size, are nearly as heavy, and need a similar loading for speedy boiling. (It is not always understood that an electric kettle is the quickest way of boiling water.) As long as the electric element is covered, the kettle need not be filled each time it is used.

Within the last few years, however, a new design of kettle has become

Figure 2.15: Electric Kettles

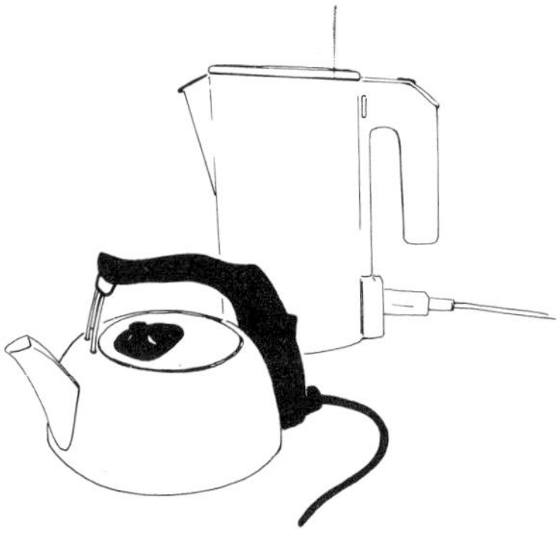

popular. This is a narrow, upright jug shape, usually made of a tough, heat-proof plastic which does not get too hot to the touch. The small element has a similar loading to the conventional shape but, because of its smaller diameter, can boil as little as one cupful of water. If filled to its maximum capacity of 1.5 litres (3 pints), it is possible to pour one or two cupfuls from it without lifting it — just by tipping it where it stands. These kettles usually have thick, easy-to-hold handles, and can be filled through the spout, without removing the lid. A 1 litre (2 pint) size is also available.

An alternative to the free-standing electric kettle, often liked by some disabled people, is the wall mounted kettle or water-boiler. This type can be mounted near the sink, and is filled from the tap through a short hose. It whistles when it boils and switches off. By carefully positioning the swivel-arm outlet and the teapot or saucepan on the draining-board or work top, no lifting is involved. Before buying, try to check that you can manage the controls and filling hose.

A variation of this is the slightly larger self-contained sink water-heater. It heats sufficient water for washing-up and, because it is plumbed into the mains, can also be used to fill a kettle for tea, which then requires only a few seconds to boil.

Tea Makers

Automatic tea makers, based on a small automatic electric kettle, may be considered a luxury, but a number of people find that they provide the necessary impetus to help them get up gradually. They can be left ready bedside the bed, complete with water, tea, milk and sugar; they incorporate an alarm clock and can be set to make the tea, then wake the sleeper up at the desired time. Some have a separate tea-pot, into which the boiling water is transferred, others drop the tea into the kettle. Some models even incorporate a radio and/or bedside light. Tea makers can, of course, also be used at any time of the day, so can be useful for leaving a hot drink for someone who cannot get about.

Coffee Makers

Although most people rely on 'instant' coffee to a large extent, it is pleasant to have 'proper' coffee for special occasions and when entertaining. The percolator and the filter machine are the two main types of coffee maker, the latter becoming more popular at the expense of the former. The percolator is not unlike a kettle, but with an enclosed element at the base of the jug which holds the water. The coffee is held in a basket through which the water percolates as it boils. Strength is controlled by an automatic timer, and some keep the coffee hot after making.

For those who maintain that coffee should never actually boil, the filter coffee maker is the answer (Figure 2.16). There are several different designs, but all incorporate a reservoir in which the water is heated to just below boiling point, a container for the finely ground coffee, through which the hot water is passed, and a jug to hold the made coffee. This stands on a small heated platform which keeps the coffee hot. Sizes range from about 0.5 to 1.5 litres (1 to 3 pints). Electric coffee grinders and roasters are also available.

Heated Food Trolleys

These need not be just an adjunct to the 'hostess with the mostest', they can be useful. For 'slow movers' they can take the worry out of trying to serve a meal on time or keeping all the dishes hot as they are cooked. They consist of a heated cupboard to hold the food, and some form of heated containers on top. The whole trolley can be pushed from kitchen to dining-room (Figure 2.17a).

Heated trays are smaller versions of the trolleys (Figure 2.17b and c). They stand on the dining table and keep food hot during service.

Figure 2.16: Filter Coffee Maker

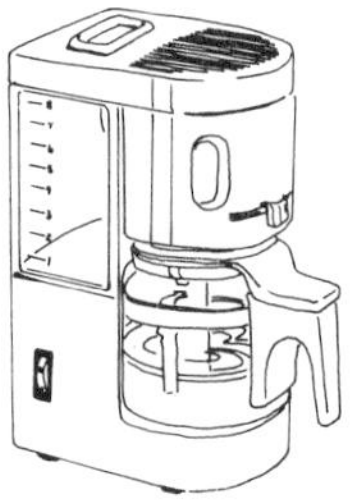

Figure 2.17: (a) Heated Food Trolley; (b), (c) Heated Food Trays

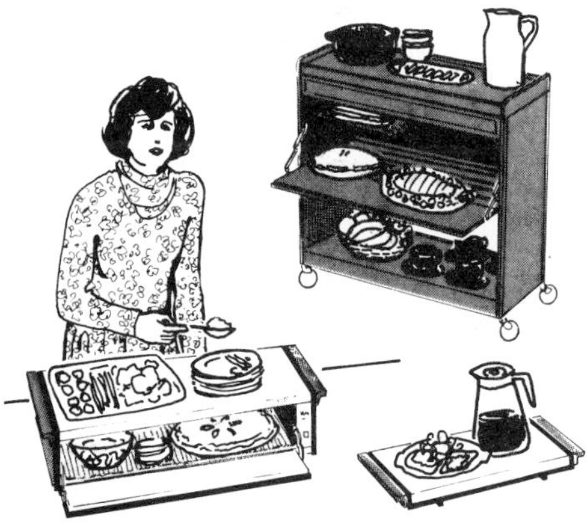

Food Mixers

Food mixers are perhaps the most versatile appliances and are found in something like half the homes in the UK. They fall into three main groups: (1) the original food mixer or food preparation machine, consisting of two beaters and a bowl, with or without other attachments; (2) the blender which developed from one of the most popular attachments, the liquidiser; (3) the new 'processor'.

All cope with routine, tedious and 'fiddling' kitchen jobs very quickly and efficiently, but they vary in which jobs they do best. Food mixers appeal to cake-makers and bread-bakers as they cope with mixing ingredients for cakes, making pastry and kneading yeast doughs. The very large ones are useful for families and have a wide choice of attachments for doing jobs such as peeling potatoes, mincing meat, making cream and slicing vegetables. But they are a good deal heavier than the smaller models which have fewer attachments. The best middle course is to choose a light food mixer plus one or more of the specialised free-standing attachments, according to need, and consider the ease of dismantling and washing them up.

Blenders

These consist simply of a large goblet with small stainless steel cutters at the base. Of 0.5 to 1 litre capacity, they quickly liquidise fruit for a variety of desserts and vegetables for soup. They also make breadcrumbs, grate cheese, chop nuts, grind coffee and mix batters, sauces and mayonnaise.

Processors

More recently, a range of more sophisticated high speed food preparation machines has appeared on the market. Called 'food processors', they work on the principle of large ultra-sharp steel blades spinning within a squat, tough plastic goblet (Figure 2.18). This is mounted above or beside a powerful motor with variable speed; the advantage of those units with the bowl beside the motor being that less shoulder movement is needed to move food from the worktop to the top of the processor. The goblets vary in shape but all have lids, without which they cannot be switched on. (Some are turned on and off with the funnel on the lid and sometimes there are separate switches.) All can hold reasonable quantities of food, but larger quantities may need to be processed in two or three batches. These machines are so quick, however, that this is not really a disadvantage. They are particularly good for slicing and shredding vegetables, for salads and for making chips, and can cope with almost any food preparation job in the kitchen so are a boon for people with limited hand or arm movement, sensitive skin or poor grip. As they vary in design, a visit to a department store where several different models are displayed would, if possible, be a distinct advantage. Again, consider the relative ease of dismantling blades,

Figure 2.18: Food Processor

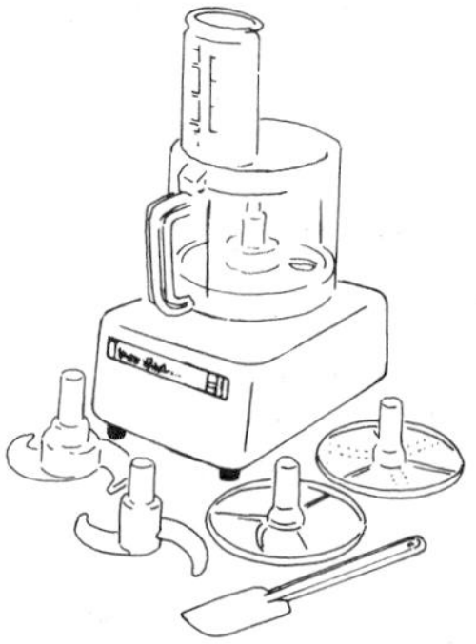

bowl and attachments, and washing them up. Care is needed when washing up all these appliances, especially by visually impaired people.

Can Openers

Electric can openers can be wall-fixed, free-standing or attachments to the largest food mixing machines. Most take several different shapes of can and, once the cans are in position, they cut the lid right off, leaving a clean edge, and hold the lid on a magnet so it does not fall into the can. Some need two hands to operate, but others can be managed with one hand. Some need more pressure than others to operate the on/off lever. (Manually operated openers are described in Chapter 3, p. 66.)

Carving Knives

Electric knives may look a little unwieldy, but once one has become accustomed to the different 'feel' and balance of them, they are easy and safe to use. All types have a finger-switch which must be held on during use; this may be difficult for some to master.

The blade is really two fine steel serrated blades operating backwards and forwards at high speed. Remember not to exert pressure — just to guide the knife and let it do the cutting. The skilled carver may take a while to get used to it, but most people will find it does a superior job for carving meat, slicing bread, cutting cake and for dealing with slippery things such as tomatoes.

Care should be taken when using with a spiked cutting board, as the spikes could damage the blade. These knives may be difficult for a person with a hand tremor to use.

Yoghurt, Cream Cheese and Ice Cream Makers, Egg Boilers

Perhaps all these come into the luxury bracket, but if a disabled person adores yoghurt or ice cream, a machine to take the hard work out of making them at home could be a blessing as well as saving time and money.

The yoghurt and cream cheese machines operate at a very low steady heat, producing between 0.5 and 1 litre of mixture at a time, made to the recipes supplied with the appliance. Those that make yoghurt in several small pots may be more convenient than the large capacity containers.

Ice cream makers are intended to hold the prepared mix made to recipes supplied with them, and have a small motor which drives paddles to stir the ice cream as it freezes, inside either the freezer or the frozen food section of a refrigerator. They have very slim flexes which run through the door of the freezer to a nearby 13amp socket outlet.

Egg boilers cook eggs perfectly every time and may be easier to handle than a saucepan and spoon if you have a hand tremor.

Lack of space may prevent you from having all the appliances you would like, but try and get personal priorities right, and add gradually to your kitchen. Fortunately, a lot of these small helpers make good presents, so a few strategically dropped hints might help!

Refrigerators and Freezers

Refrigerators

Now accepted as an essential part of every kitchen, the refrigerator usually takes the place of the old pantry or larder, especially in small homes and flats. There is a wide choice of models, both electric and gas, to suit most people's needs.

The purpose of a refrigerator is to store food for a given length of time in such a condition as to prevent the growth of bacteria; modern refrigerators have a compartment for keeping commercially frozen food for a longer period of time depending on the star marking. Waste caused by poor storage facilities can be reduced and this ultimately means saving money: an average-sized domestic refrigerator uses about one unit of electricity per day.

Meals can be planned and shopped for days ahead, and dishes prepared beforehand, thus saving time and last minute rush. If a visitor brings a prepared dish it can be stored safely overnight.

Some models offer the choice of push-button or semi-automatic defrosting, and a few have fully automatic defrosting. Some also show a number of modern extras, such as an ice-cube store or a drinks dispenser, which may solve personal handling difficulty.

A refrigerator in the home offers its user a high degree of independence because it keeps perishable food safe for a reasonable time, and can help in forward meal preparation for a day or two in advance. But it should never be regarded as a long-term food store, as food will still 'go off' in a refrigerator, but more slowly.

The following points must be considered.

1. Have the right-sized refrigerator for your needs. For minimum space allow approximately 28 litres (1 cubic foot) per person plus one. If you live alone, the smallest floor-standing refrigerator (about 84 litres/3 cu ft) is ideal, as it is a good policy to get one larger than 'adequate'. Sizes vary from 84 litres (3 cu ft) to about 336 litres (12 cu ft). One very small refrigerator (28 litres/1 cu ft of storage) can be wall-hung or stood on a worktop, but if you have room, the larger ones are better value for money.
2. Think how much you are going to use the frozen food storage compartment which will keep frozen food for up to three months (Figure 2.19). Two-door refrigerators have the frozen food compartment separated from the main cabinet which means that the opening of the refrigerator does not interfere with the temperature of the frozen food compartment. Others have a separate freezer compartment in which small amounts of food can be frozen and frozen food stored.
3. The shape of the refrigerator you choose will depend on the amount of floor space available and whether you need to use the top as a work surface. Small refrigerators can be wall-hung or put on work surfaces or plinths, or built in to specially designed kitchen units.
4. It is important that the door should open easily, so decide whether you

Figure 2.19: Star-marking Chart

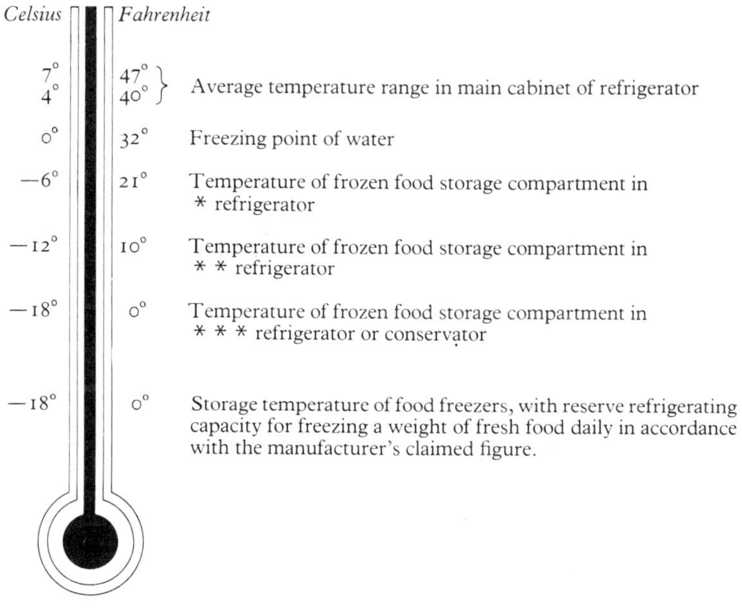

Source: The Electricity Council

want a left- or right-opening door, according to your kitchen plan — some models give a choice of opening. Almost all refrigerators have magnetic door seals and require very little effort to open; always try before you buy.
5. The internal arrangement of the refrigerator varies with each model. Make sure you can manage the salad drawer and that the dairy fitments in the door are stable. Check that the door to the frozen food compartment is easy to open and whether it will stay open while you get something out.
6. Decide whether you can cope with the defrosting of a refrigerator. (Could you handle the drip tray with water in it?) If not, choose a self-defrosting model. (See 'Using the refrigerator', Chapter 3, p. 84).

Pay a visit to your local gas or electricity premises if possible before deciding on a model, and check on servicing arrangements.

Storage of Food in the Refrigerator

Each manufacturer advises on this but the following general rules apply:

1. everything must be clean;
2. food must be cooled quickly before being put inside, otherwise the warmth or steam will cause rapid frost built-up. Do this by leaving covered food containers in a cool place or in a bowl of cold water until they have stopped steaming;
3. all food must be covered to prevent dehydration and absorption of flavour and smells, for instance, melon, fish or foods containing garlic;
4. part-used frozen food must be covered and returned to the refrigerator as quickly as possible, and used as fresh food.

Freezers

It is essential to have a freezer for long-term food storage, in addition to using canned and dehydrated foodstuffs. The ownership of these appliances has expanded rapidly in the last decade, so that now well over half the homes in the UK have one, and some may feel they are essential for disabled people. Certainly they have a number of advantages.
1. Staple food, for instance, bread, meat, fish, vegetables and fruit can always be available. Anyone who cooks in large quantities (bread, cakes or casseroles, for example) can freeze the surplus for future needs or 'bad' days.
2. Fruits and vegetables in season, when they are cheaper or available from the garden, can be frozen and stored.
3. Shopping can be done less frequently (it may be necessary to adjust budgets from weekly to monthly).
4. A food freezer can be kept anywhere cool and dry and where there is a suitable socket outlet.
5. Money can be saved by buying economy packs and using a little at a time.

6. Nutritional values are in no way affected by freezing.
7. 'Left-overs' from a meal can be frozen for another day.

Owners of microwave cookers find these two appliances together make for very easy meal preparation. Before buying a freezer, try to read one or two of the numerous books on the subject. Full manufacturer's instructions are issued with each one. Anyone buying a freezer should decide in advance if he or she is able to undertake the simple wrapping and labelling procedures essential for good results, because the freezer can be twice as useful to those who are able to keep home produced food in the freezer as well as some of the excellent ready-frozen commercial foods.

A freezer needs to be defrosted two or three times a year. As this can entail quite a lot of effort in removing and replacing the food, it may be as well to seek help for this job, and to do it when stocks are fairly low.

Chest freezers should be defrosted about once or twice a year. Upright freezers may need defrosting two or three times. Choose a time when the contents are at a minimum. *Always study the manufacturer's defrosting instructions as different models require different methods.*

In general:

1. some hours before defrosting, put plenty of newspapers and an old, clean blanket into the freezer so that they become thoroughly chilled;
2. switch off the electricity, and transfer the remaining food to a cold place. Stack the packets closely together, wrap them in several layers of the chilled newspaper and cover them with the chilled blanket;
3. leave the freezer open, and place bowls of hot water inside it. As soon as the ice has loosened, remove it by scraping down the sides of the freezer with a blunt spatula of wood or plastic. Never use a metal instrument;
4. spread a towel on the bottom of the cabinet to catch the ice so that it can be removed easily;
5. finally, wash the walls of the cabinet with hand-hot water in which a little bicarbonate of soda has been dissolved. Allow the walls to dry thoroughly before closing the lid or door;
6. switch on the electricity and return the food to the cabinet immediately.

Early freezers were usually 'chests' which were sometimes difficult to reach into. Most freezers are now upright cabinets similar to a medium refrigerator, and it is possible to get matching pairs of these two appliances, each about 150 litres (5 cu ft) in size. In this case, the refrigerator part (called a 'larder fridge') does not have a separate frozen food section, as ice can be made and food stored in the freezer. Some have shelves or baskets which can be drawn out.

Fridge-freezers

These appliances, which combine both appliances in one cabinet with two

Figure 2.20: Fridge-freezer

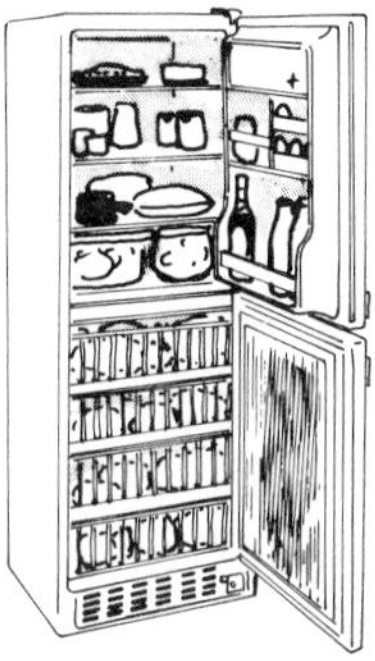

doors, are very practical (Figure 2.20). They can have both halves of similar capacity or a big fridge and small freezer or *vice versa*; and either the fridge or freezer (usually the latter) can be at the bottom. Consider these alternatives carefully before buying to ensure that you can easily reach the half you are likely to use most. Wheelchair-users or very short people may prefer two separate units set side-by-side on the floor, or on shallow plinths.

Although, ideally, a freezer should be in a cool dry site, it is usually more convenient to have it in the kitchen where it can be readily reached. For this reason, a disabled user may well consider it worth the slightly higher running costs entailed in keeping the freezer or fridge-freezer in the kitchen. An upright freezer uses approximately one-and-a-half to one-and-three-quarters units per cubic foot per week or one unit for every 15 litres per week.

Dishwashers

Dishwashers have been on the market for many years, in a variety of sizes and types. Somehow, they have never caught the fancy of British people, and yet they are probably the greatest home helps of all. Washing-up is something we all have to do every day, sometimes three or four times a day, yet only one in 20 homes has a dishwasher; washing clothes may be done only once or twice a week, yet 16 out of 20 homes own a washing machine! However, for people with many kinds of disablement they are invaluable; for people with skin conditions caused or worsened by allergy to soaps, powders or washing-up liquids, they are almost essential to lessen contact with those irritants. Visually handicapped users can have confidence that all their crockery will be really clean.

Most dishwashers are floor-standing but some smaller table-top models will stand on the draining board. Even so, these cost almost as much as some of the bigger ones, and as the larger ones can take so many more items, they are probably a better bet. Small families can easily rinse and stack dishes in the machine, ready for one good wash-up once the machine is full. Although this means that a few more cups and plates may be needed in use, it is usually more economical in the long run. Sizes are quoted in 'place settings' — three to four place settings for small machines; ten to 14 for full-size models.

Inside trays vary slightly in arrangement, and it is a good idea when buying a new machine to take a small selection of everyday dishes, including a dinner plate, to see if they fit in easily. Modern dishwashers clean most pots, pans, china and cutlery, but it is worth remembering that there are some items, such as lead crystal and bone-handled knives, which should not be machine-washed. Several china and cutlery manufacturers now indicate that their goods are machine-washable.

Laundry Appliances

Laundry appliances are included in this section because only a very small percentage of British homes have room for them elsewhere. For most people, the days when the laundry used to be sent out are gone, so that this somewhat exhausting job has to be done at home. Modern, easy-care textiles which are easy to wash and dry and need little or no ironing have eased the situation (and it is wise to dispense with 'family heirloom' bed linen and table-linen, for instance, to save energy). The excellent modern detergents — formulated for use with new fabrics and appliances — should be used strictly according to instructions for best results; sufferers from allergic and other skin conditions should be guided further in their use by their doctor.

Sometimes older people feel it behoves them to continue to wash clothes by hand, on the principle of 'if it was good enough for my mother, it is good enough for me'. But surely most of our mothers would have jumped at the chance of reducing heavy laundry work had they had the facilities of this generation? Others may argue that now the family is grown up, the smaller amount of washing for one or two people can be done by hand. But the amount of household linen is still considerable, and disabled and older people should seriously consider buying a washing machine.

Automatic Washing Machines

These machines are by far the best solution for disabled people. Once the clothes and washing powders are put into the machine and the controls set, the whole procedure — soaking, washing, rinsing and spin-drying — is carried out automatically. A considerable range of machines, at varying prices, is available on the market (Figure 2.21). Some of the most expen-

Figure 2.21: Automatic Washing Machine

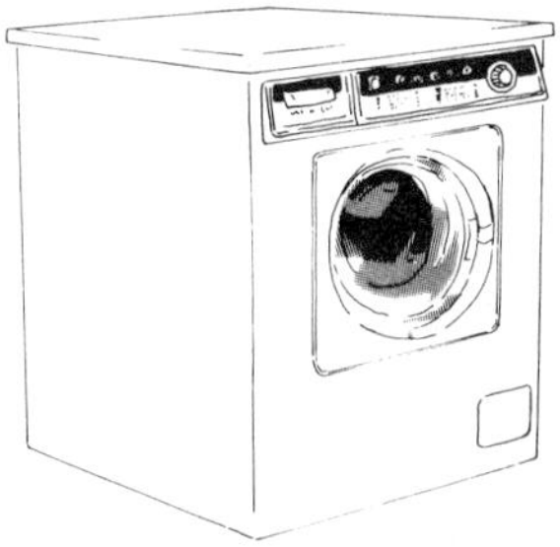

sive have very sophisticated features which are not always necessary, but it may not be sensible to buy the cheapest, bearing in mind that a few more pounds may buy a helpful labour-saving 'extra' for the disabled user. The new electronically controlled machines are simple to use and very reliable.

Most automatic washing machines are loaded through a door in the front, so are easy to use from a sitting position. Some of these have the controls at the front also; others have them at the back, and it is wise to check that they can be both reached and seen by the user. For people who cannot bend, there are one or two machines which can be loaded from the top.

Several manufacturers offer alternative sets of controls for blind users on some machines. Most knobs are easy to handle.

Single and Twintub Machines

Although they have automatic features, these machines usually demand more of the operator, but some older people prefer this. However, operating them does entail, at some stage, the lifting of heavy, wet clothes. Twintub machines incorporate efficient spin-dryers.

For those who have only very few 'smalls' to wash weekly, or who prefer to wash by hand, a separate spin-dryer is invaluable.

Tumble Dryers

Tumble dryers are just about essential for mothers with babies and other children, flat-dwellers and anyone who cannot get out to hang clothes. Indeed, hanging clothes outside to dry is a needless labour these days for anyone. For those who insist on 'a good blow', revolving clothes-lines and electric 'rain alarms' can sometimes ease the difficulties.

Irons

Ironing is much easier these days, too. Towels, tea-towels, polycotton bed-linen and underclothes do not need ironing. Easycare shirts, dresses and blouses need only touching-up with a light iron. Modern irons are light-

Figure 2.22: Iron

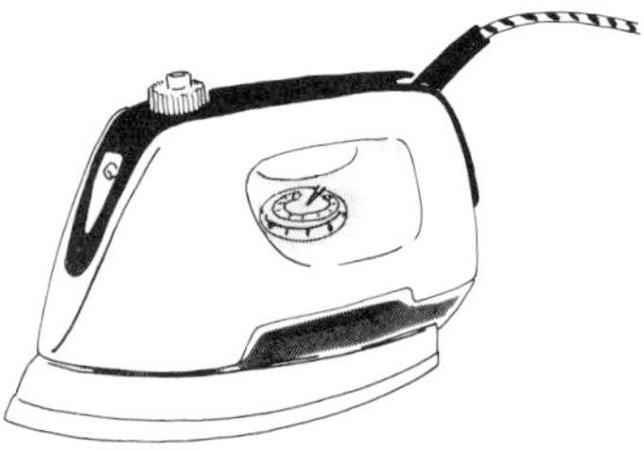

weight, have thermostatic controls geared to the International Laundry Code Symbols and tapered points to get into corners (Figure 2.22). Most of these have easily felt controls, or can be brailled. Some have central flexes, and others can be adjusted when bought, to be suitable for either a left or right-handed user. Adjustable ironing boards and heat reflecting board covers make the job even easier.

3 Coping with Problems

Marian Lane

The worst problem that many disabled people have to cope with in the kitchen is the *thought* that they may be unable to cope. This thought also worries other members of the family, as well as friends and far-flung relations. In many cases, a complete re-think about methods, equipment and kitchen layout is needed. However, most people do find their own way of coping. Some say, 'Oh, it's just common sense', but on closer questioning, you find that they have, in fact, either altered their routine or chosen more suitable equipment; they might, for example, have split preparation and cooking time, have bought very lightweight or double-handled saucepans, new kitchen units with rounded edges and 'D' handles, or be lost without their own special sharp knife.

Hospital rehabilitation departments can offer the opportunity to try new methods and different equipment, so ask the doctor to refer you as an out-patient if you think you would benefit from practising new methods. Appendix I gives details about people and organisations who offer help of many kinds.

It is worth taking time to try out new items of equipment. Ask the shop assistant if you can handle anything you think might be useful. Look in the kitchenware sections of big stores which carry large stocks of different manufacturer's goods. To be worth having, a piece of equipment should make your life easier or even enable you to do something you would otherwise be unable to do; buying an electric food mixer, for example, might give you time and energy to do other things. In the end, one or two small changes may be all that are needed.

Individuals differ greatly in their enthusiasm for cooking and the amount of effort they are prepared to put in to resolve a problem. This chapter, rather than listing solutions for people with different types of disability, sets out a great many different ideas and methods for coping with particular difficulties. All of the ideas and items have been tried and found useful.

One very important point: you may feel at first that you need many more adaptations and aids in the kitchen than are in fact necessary, and finish up with a kitchen full of equipment you don't use. Think carefully before deciding what you need to suit your lifestyle, and keep the equipment as simple as possible. Some items of equipment are simpler and more efficient to use than others. The basic points to consider when choosing equipment are versatility, durability, easy maintenance and cheapness; but it is advisable to go through the detailed check list in the section 'Choosing Equipment' (p. 60) each time.

Practice with existing equipment, plus a rearrangement of the kitchen may be all that is necessary to ease the workload.

Conserving Energy

Plan both the kitchen and the work so that the least physical effort is required: for disabled people with limited strength, it is even more important to save energy on the basic day-to-day tasks so that there is some to spare for enjoyment. In addition, it may be possible to time the tasks so that they can be done at the point in the day when energy is at its highest. When considering your own situation, the following check list may be helpful.

1. Planning saves work:

(a) plan a week's menus at the beginning of the week and make your shopping list from it to cover the week ahead (but see also Chapter 6, p. 119);

(b) if possible, do your main shopping weekly, but try to get out as often as possible for items like fresh vegetables;

(c) store the implements you need near where the job will be done;

(d) collect all tools/ingredients before you start;

(e) store food, if possible, ready prepared to save time when cooking; for instance, cut up the meat, wash greens, scrub carrots, chop parsley. Store for short periods in covered containers or polythene bags in the fridge. Rubbed-in pastry or scone mix will keep, ready for water or milk to be added when wanted. In this way it is possible to prepare food when you feel like it (there may be times in the day or 'off days' when you don't);

(f) some people who feel at their most energetic in the mornings could use a slow cooker (see Chapter 2, p. 39), preparing the evening meal in the morning, allowing it to cook all day so that it is ready for eating at suppertime. Some gas cookers have a slow setting which can be used in a similar way or automatic controls could be set to turn on the meal at a later time in the day;

(g) keep your equipment well maintained so that it is efficient; for instance, make sure that knives and scissors are sharp.

2. Make sure you are comfortable and steady before you start work. Ideally, the working surface should be at a height so that, as you work, your hands are about level with your waist. If you have weak arms you will probably find it easier to work at a lower level (on a level with your hands when they are by your sides), to minimise the need to raise the arms and put the hands in a position where the arm and body weight can be used for any pressure needed (using the bottom of the sink as a work surface may be a help).

If possible, have different heights available for either standing or sitting (easily adjustable cantilever tables, for instance, which also have space underneath for knees). Someone who relies on a walking stick in the house should fit a clip to the work top or trolley to keep the stick out of the way and readily available (while someone in a wheelchair may choose to work on a tray on their lap). A useful alternative is to fix a coat hook with a sticky back to the kitchen wall or unit so that the stick can be put on this to prevent it falling on the floor.

3. Try to push or slide, instead of lifting, heavy items. This will be made easier if there are work surfaces beside the cooker and the sink is level with both. If they are not level, you could have a small ramp made out of lino, vinyl and/or a strip of wood to put beside the cooker, or use a trolley. (See also 'Carrying things' on p. 90). However, remember that pans should not be pulled across ceramic hobs, which are easily scratched.

4. Never stand when you can sit. Some people prefer a stool with a back for stability (Figure 3.1), some like one that can be moved about, while others feel safer on a non-mobile stool with a sloping seat (Figure 3.2). If possible, have two stools, of different heights, for different jobs. Swivel office chairs can be turned from side to side without the sitter having to rise, while the Tendex chair, especially designed for disabled people, has a wide stable base, although you must take into account the amount of floor space occupied by such a chair (Figure 3.3). Some special stools are sprung under the seat which then tilts with the sitter as he or she stands, to exert an extra push (Figure 3.4). A brake fitted in a moving chair is more expensive, but it is a useful addition. A chair (with a back) on castors (such as the Mayfair Glideabout) is one useful solution and is obtainable with brakes (Figure 3.5). Some people use office-type chairs with castors for mobility, pushing themselves around with their feet or pulling on the furniture; constant getting up and down is therefore avoided. However, care must be

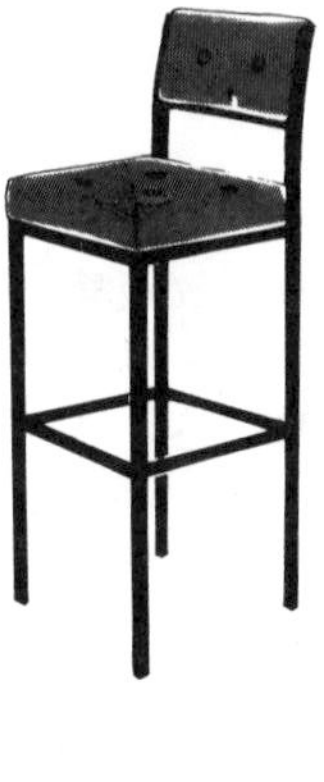

Figure 3.1: High Stool with Back

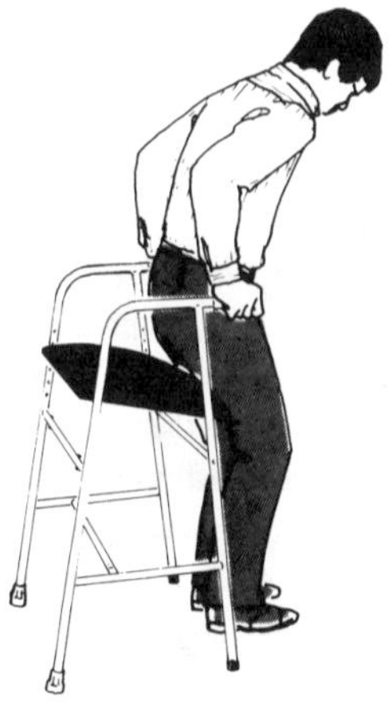

Figure 3.2: Hayman Perching Stool

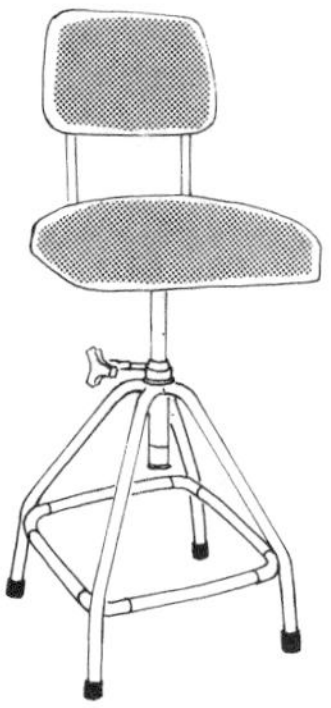

Figure 3.3: Swivel Chair with Wide Base

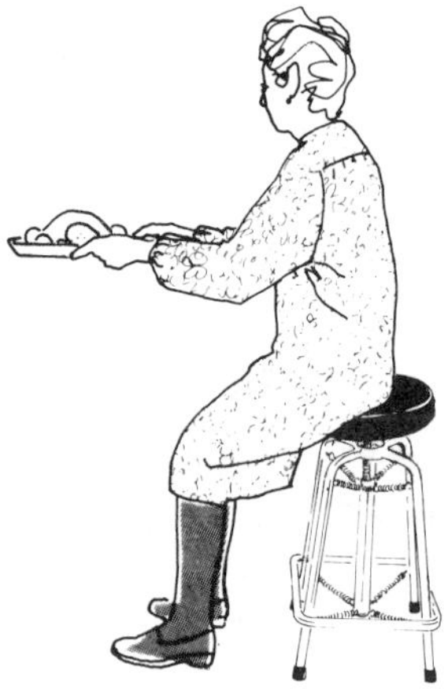

Figure 3.4: Floating Stool: Spring under Seat

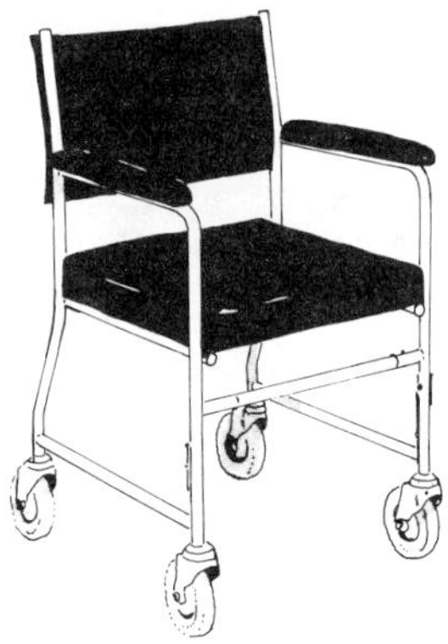

Figure 3.5: Mayfair Glideabout

taken when getting in and out of this type of chair as it could easily run away and leave the sitter on the floor. If possible, the chair should be backed against something solid (a wall or unit) before sitting down or getting up.

5. Someone who stands to work at the sink should make sure, if there is room, that there is a suitable chair nearby to rest on.

6. Allow time for doing the job — usually longer than you think!

7. Consider using convenience foods occasionally: sliced bread, canned food, dried vegetables, ready-cooked meat, fish and chips, packet cake mixes. Boil-in-the-bag food is also very useful; for instance, fish in sauce,

rice and stews. If opening such foods is a problem, look at different ideas for opening packs (see pp. 65-8). Frozen foods, although sometimes more expensive, can save a great deal of preparation — especially the ready-prepared individual meals. The extra cost is also offset by lack of waste.

8. If you have a freezer, it is useful to bake twice as much as usual (or more when you are feeling energetic) so that the excess can be stored in the freezer ready for a lazy day or one when energy is being expended on some other activity. Soups, stews, cooked meat, steamed puddings, pies and tarts as well as cakes and biscuits can also be stored (see Chapter 2, p. 50 on how to use the freezer).

In conjunction with points 7 and 8, consider purchasing a microwave cooker (especially one with a defrost facility) which cooks food quickly and is easy to use (see Chapter 2, p. 40). A microwave cooker is particularly useful for very severely disabled people who often need to heat up (easily and safely) food which has been previously prepared for them by others.

9. Use one-stage cake, sauce, pastry and bread recipes.

10. Try to organise the kitchen so that you do not have to carry anything a long distance; a trolley and/or hatch to the eating area can be useful.

11. Save carrying by eating in the kitchen if possible, and keep a teapot, kettle and teabags in the living room for tea-breaks.

12. Avoid planning a menu that involves last minute preparation for more than one course, especially a 'party' menu.

Fatigue

Everyone needs to assess for themselves how long they can remain at one task, and which tasks they find the most tiring. Fatigue will probably accentuate symptoms and can therefore be frightening.

Try not to begin an activity that cannot be put on one side halfway through. Most people are quick to learn how long they can work before they need a rest, but do not be too ambitious in the meantime. Learning new methods can be very tiring and frustrating, but practice really will improve performance. On the other hand, it can be a mistake to be too careful as enough exercise should be taken to maintain mobility.

Choosing Equipment

Before buying any equipment, whether large or small, it is wise to consider first the four elementary precepts of good design.

1. Does it work?
2. Will it give value for money?
3. Do you like the look and feel of it?
4. Can you operate the equipment without help?

Then you can proceed to make a more detailed analysis as to whether the equipment works in the way that suits you best, and whether it fits into your particular kitchen. The following check list will help you to choose the right equipment, and to eliminate unnecessary items.

1. Why do you want it? Would something else double up?
2. Can you afford it, or can you get help to obtain it? (See Chapter 1, p. 4)
3. Does it do a job you would otherwise find difficult, painful, tiring, time-consuming or impossible?
4. Will it be accommodated easily in the space available (and is there an accessible electric socket if the equipment requires one)? It may be necessary to rearrange the kitchen or to get rid of something else to make room for the new purchase.
5. Is handling it (that is, getting it out of the cupboard, from under the sink, lifting it from the shelf) within your capabilities, particularly as regards weight?
6. Can you operate it without difficulty? Before buying the equipment think through the whole cycle of use in the situation where it would be used. Is every stage possible for you? Could any stage of operation be omitted?
7. Is it stable?
8. Can you operate and turn the handle if there is one? (A lever or bar type is easiest for most weak hands.)
9. If there is a lid, can you lift it? A large knob is easier.
10. Are the markings on the controls visible to you?
11. Is it easy to clean after use? Does it need dismantling to clean it and, if so, can you manage this easily?
12. Can you reach and turn the knobs or switches?
13. Does it require the minimum of attention (that is, renewal of batteries, emptying waste, topping up of fluid)? Could you manage this job?
14. Are servicing facilities readily available? This is a most important point as difficulty in servicing could render the purchase of large appliances worthless.
15. If you are visually handicapped, does the colour of the piece of equipment (chopping board, for example) contrast well with the work surface?

If the answer to all these questions is 'yes' — go ahead and buy the equipment! Many shopkeepers and assistants are willing, if asked, to demonstrate equipment and allow the potential customer to try using it. See also 'Choosing a cooker', Chapter 2, p. 36.

Colour Contrast

Choosing equipment in contrasting colours or in colours that contrast with the working surface can be of great help to people with poor sight. For example, if utensils with dark handles are bought, the handles will stand out against a light work surface or *vice versa.* The work surface should be plain, not patterned.

A chopping board with one dark side can be used for chopping onions, for example, while the other light side, can be used for chopping or slicing brightly coloured vegetables such as tomatoes or beetroot.

These ideas can be combined. If a worktop has light and dark sections, for example, it will be easier to see spills on it (flour on the dark surface, dirty smudges on the light one).

Storage and Labelling

Hints on Labelling

If you cannot see labels clearly, try one of the following ideas.

1. Use large dymo tape; when stuck on, the raised lettering can be felt. Kits are available from stationers, and the tape can be obtained in a variety of bright colours.
2. Also available from stationers are the self-adhesive raised letters for larger items.
3. Toy magnetic letters or elastic bands round articles can be used as a coding system on, for example, cans in store.
4. Black waterproof marker pens, available in a range of thicknesses, make clear markings on cans, jars and boxes.
5. The RNIB have a range of helpful aids including: a tube of 'Hi Mark' which, if squeezed like toothpaste, can make raised marks — script, braille, or Moon — in bright orange on almost anything, such as wood, paper, metal, non-woven cloth, plastic; and a range of brailled labels, for instance, hook-on, stick-on and magnetic.

Finally, however you choose to label your stores, do it as soon as you get them home and, to save time and energy, keep the labelling kit together in one place.

Hints on Storage

1. If you have sliding doors on your cupboards, a plastic stop can be fitted to the door on the inner track to prevent one disappearing behind the other.
2. If space inside permits, a shelf can be fitted to the back of a cupboard door that opens outwards, as long as the door hinges are strong enough and there is a raised edge on the shelf to prevent things falling off. Alternatively, put hooks on the back of the door, and hang bags on them for, say, cleaning materials. Metal baskets, string bags and plastic carriers hung on the back of a door will also hold things.

3. A door on the cupboard is not essential and can be removed if it is really inconvenient. Open shelving is useful, but since it can quickly get dirty and greasy, it is wise to use open shelves mainly for objects in daily use.

4. If you cannot reach the back of your shelves, put a strip of wood on the shelf to prevent the drift of cans to the back.

5. A sliding plastic basket may be fitted under a shelf for small jars and spices.

6. Mini-drawers screw under a shelf — small plastic drawers with easy-to-grasp handles; others hang on the shelf with wire supports.

7. Plates are easier to reach if they are stored vertically in a plastic washing-up rack or in a plastic-covered record-holder-type rack.

8. 'Space savers' (plastic-covered wire shelves and racks) stand on a work top or cupboard shelf to subdivide it, or may be fixed on to the wall or back of a door.

9. Plastic cutlery trays are also useful for kitchen tools and keep a drawer more organised.

10. Plastic oblong vegetable racks can stand on a small floor space.

11. Small mobile vegetable racks are versatile and can be moved about as you work.

12. Plastic-covered, adjustable shelf systems for the wall are easy to put up.

13. A system of drawers or baskets, each on runners, in a unit can replace conventional closed-in drawers.

14. Tools and small utensils can hang on hooks on a plain or a peg board.

15. Rotating shelves in a cupboard (or small turntables on a shelf) bring any item on the shelf close to hand without stretching (Figure 3.6). See also Chapter 1, p. 14.

Figure 3.6: Two-tier Roundabout

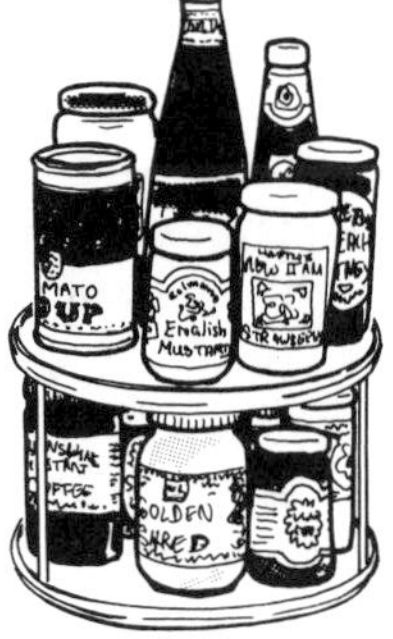

Preparation of Food

Holding and Steadying

One-handed people obviously need to be able to fix the object they are working with, but most people's safety, efficiency and comfort can be improved if they are able to steady what they are doing without having to keep a tight hold on it. This applies particularly to those who have weak grip, are unsteady or shaky or who tire easily.

Slip-resistant Materials. These are placed under a bowl, chopping board or pan to stop it slipping while you work. Examples include:

1. Dycem is a sticky plastic material, probably the most slip-resistant available. It is produced as mats in various shapes and sizes or can be bought by the metre, and in the form of netting. Dust and dirt make this material less efficient, but washing in hot water will rectify this and will not destroy its slip-resistant property;
2. any damp cloth will help prevent slipping when placed between the utensil and work surface. A sponge dishcloth is the most efficient. It can also be used to create a contrast between bowl and work surface if contrasting china is not available;
3. plastic foam sheeting can be used in the same way as above;
4. double suction cups and suction soap holders (see 'Mixing', p. 75).

Aids for Holding Things. There is a wide range of these aids.

1. Some people find screw clamps indispensable for fixing boards and tools. However, some worktops are unsuitable for clamps; for instance, those that are flush with the side of a cupboard and have no rim, are too deep, or are not strong enough to withstand the damage that constant clamping will inevitably cause. Some aids have a clamp incorporated in their design, so this needs to be considered when choosing. Some of the specially designed clamps have an easy screwing mechanism: one clamp has optional interchangeable grips enabling it to hold different-shaped items.

The Orange Aids System consists of a series of clamping devices designed to stabilise a wide range of utensils. It may be useful in the kitchen to stabilise graters, whisks and jars, for example.

2. The Bellyclamp hooks onto the work surface; the grip on the item to be held is maintained by the user pushing against the clamp with stomach or hip. This obviates the need for nuts and bolts in any of the operations required.
3. Bulldog clips are useful for holding or weighting light objects (often books or leaflets) or as a closure for a polythene bag.
4. Spring clothes pegs can be used as above and require less effort to open.

Other aids for holding things include:
5. bowl holders (see 'Mixing' p. 75);
6. pan handle holders (see 'Using Cooker Hob' p. 79);
7. spike-boards for holding vegetables (see 'Peeling' p. 68); and
8. aids for holding bread for cutting and buttering and holding meat for slicing (see p. 72).

Opening Jars/Bottles/Cans

Opening Jars. The wide range of aids available from household stores to help people to undo screw tops fall into the following categories:

1. the V-grip — either hand-held or screwed to the underside of a shelf (Figure 3.7). The jar top is pushed between the arms of the V until it wedges tightly enough to hold it for turning. With the fixed model, the jar is then turned clockwise to loosen the top. Some hand-held models can also open lever-tops (Figure 3.8), and some have a lid piercer;
2. a handle with a thong or a steel band at one end that can be tightened around the lid of the jar, so that the handle can be used as a lever. These aids generally need both hands to operate them;
3. a cone-shaped rubber cap with a fluted surface inside, to be placed over the lid to aid hand grip (Figure 3.9). It is also possible to hold the cap in the opening of the door at the hinge side and shut the door to give a firm hold; but this may dent the inner edge of the door;
4. a lever handle with adjustable clamp that slides along the handle to grip the lid for turning (Figure 3.10).

Figure 3.7: Skyline V-grip Fixes under Shelf

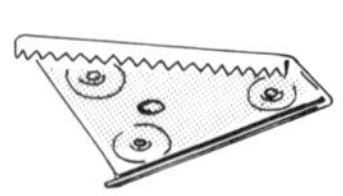

Figure 3.8: Turnaid Hand-held V-grip

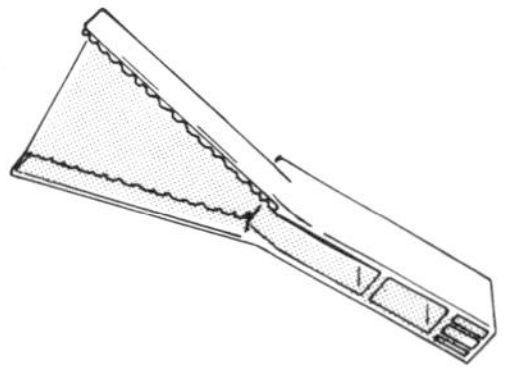

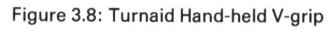

Figure 3.9: Cone-shaped Twister

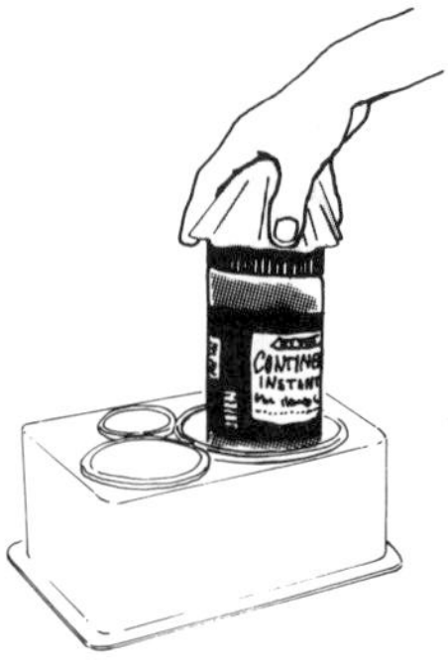

Figure 3.10: Open-all Jar Opener

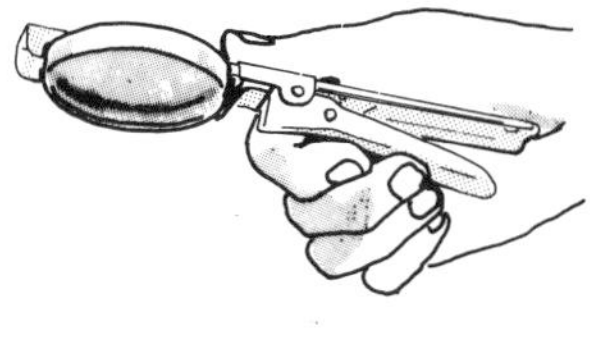

If you have none of these, try one or all of the following:

1. if a screw top is very stiff, turn the jar upside down and give the lid a couple of smart knocks on the table, either on the rim or directly onto the top (or bang the top with a rolling pin);
2. sit down and hold the jar between your knees;
3. put the jar in a drawer and hold it there with your hip as you turn the lid (take care as this may damage the surface of the drawer);
4. with a metal lid or glass top on a glass jar, rotate the lid under running hot water;
5. as a permanent measure, screw the lids of storage jars on the underside of a shelf or wall cupboard, so the jar is unscrewed from the lid, which is much easier than *vice versa.* Instant coffee jars are ideal for this;
6. wear a rubber glove for better grip.

Opening Bottles. The aids and ideas for opening screw-top bottles are the same as those for opening jars: among the types mentioned in that section, some are designed for the smaller neck of a bottle rather than a jar. One useful tip — many people use nutcrackers for opening bottles.

Wine Bottles. If the problem is only drawing the cork (that is, the cork-screw can be inserted without much trouble), several makes of corkscrew (some wooden, some metal) work by screwing the corkscrew in as usual, then reversing direction and screwing the cork out.

Alternatively, one tool pumps air into the bottle through a thin spindle pushed through the cork, and blows the cork out. The pin is easier to push in than a corkscrew but snaps fairly easily, so it needs to be handled with respect. The air must be pumped in slowly — just enough to move the cork, and not at such speed that the cork flies out (or the bottle explodes!). This tool is not recommended for any but standard-shaped bottles. If a wine cork defies removal, it can sometimes be pushed into the bottle instead, as long as you are not drinking a sparkling wine.

Opening Cans. Can-openers fall into two main categories — electrically or manually operated.

Electric openers are described in Chapter 2 (see p. 47). They are easy to operate and, with the advent of hand-held openers, can be useful for one-handed people as well as those with problems such as weak grip.

Manually operated openers come in many shapes and sizes: some are wall-fixed, others hand-held. Someone using a wall-fixed opener has to hold the can under the cutting knife while turning the handle to rotate the knife. With some models, a lever has to be pushed over the top to secure the can under the blade: with others, the can is gripped as the blade or cog-wheel begins to turn. The handles are usually small and it could be difficult to hold the can up — especially if it is large. One opener has a large square handle making it easier to grasp; it turns smoothly and the user can easily see where to place the tin, although it has no magnet to hold the tin.

Stands are available to support the can either as a part of the whole opener or as a separate item. The first cut into the can is probably the hardest part of the job for anyone unable to 'push'.

The wall-hung openers with stands are particularly helpful for one-handed people; the height of the stand can be adjusted and varies according to the model. The stand on one model is set on a central screw so that the height is adjusted by rotating the stand. This requires some skill to bring the lip of the can under the cutting knife: one way round this is to place a block of plastic foam on the tray to create a resilient base for the can. On another model, the stand has a loaded spring underneath, so that the can is pushed down on the stand and brought upwards under the blade without further adjustment. Care should be taken to keep a firm hold of the can when removing it after opening — the strong spring could deliver the contents of the can over a wide area. Another stand is adjusted by pressing a lever on a sliding mechanism underneath. This requires dexterity, and it is not easy to adjust the edge of the can under the blade.

If someone is fitting your wall opener for you, make sure it is fixed at the height most suitable for *you.*

Other manually operated openers (obviously of no use to one-handed people) include the 'butterfly' type, used by gripping the two handles together in one hand to fasten onto the can edge, and turning the 'butterfly' knob with the other hand to open it.

The sizes both of the gripping handles and the turning knob vary; the cutting 'knife' also varies between a pointed 'knife' and a cutting wheel similar to those on some of the wall-hung openers. The larger handles are generally the easiest to grip and turn. A pointed cutter is probably the best for piercing the can initially, but the wheel seems to need less pressure to complete the actual opening. As with other openers, the first cut — piercing the tin — is the hardest to make. These openers are available from household stores. Some food mixers, such as the Kenwood, have a can opener attachment.

The ordinary simple lever can-openers are probably least useful to anyone with limited use of arms and hands; one exception is the 'Waves' opener, which is available in right or left-handed models and can be used in conjunction with a clamp for one-handed people (Figure 3.11).

In addition, a small vice attached to the work top might be useful in a kitchen, especially for holding cans that are awkwardly shaped, like steak and kidney pie cans.

Information on other can-openers designed for left-handed use is available from a shop in London which has a mail order service (see Appendix II, p. 152).

Figure 3.11: Savage's Grip Clamp

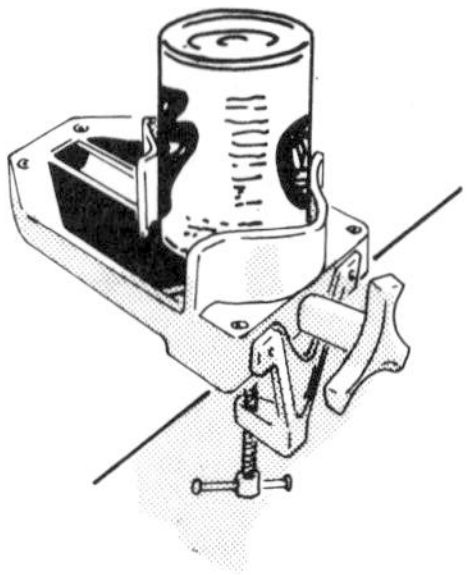

Key-opening Cans

1. It is possible to open a square can with an ordinary can-opener.
2. The ring-top type seems easier to manipulate than the 'key' type but needs a lot of tugging to open. It can help to loop the ring onto a hook on the wall. (It might be as well to tip out the oil after the first 'tug'.)
3. Cans with a key can be difficult for everyone, especially if the metal tab for the key is on the corner of the tin. Some tins have the tab on one end which is easier to control.
4. Large 'keys' can be bought at household stores and slipped out of the rolled-up lid after opening, to be used again. These are much easier to use than the small 'keys' packed with the can.
5. A skewer threaded through the 'key' loop makes a good lever for twisting.

Peeling

If it is possible to work comfortably near the sink — preferably sitting down — it will save carrying the vegetables to be washed. But first consider whether this need be attempted at all.

Ways to Avoid Peeling Potatoes. Scrub them with a brush or a plastic (not metal) pot scourer (especially effective on new potatoes). They can be boiled in their skins, as can carrots, to be peeled or not after cooking. Even quite small potatoes will bake in the oven without getting too hard if cooking oil is rubbed into their skins. A scrubbing brush attached to the sink by suction pads might prove useful for one-handed people.

Other alternatives are to use instant potato for 'mash', canned new potatoes, especially if they are roasted or used as part of a salad, or oven chips.

Peelers. Peelers divide roughly into the following groups: (1) automatic; (2) clamped to worktop; (3) hand-held with enlarged handles.

Other aids to preparing vegetables include spike boards to hold the vegetables while they are being peeled; one-handed people, especially, find these useful. (See p. 70 for more details.)

1. Automatic peelers are either electrically operated or water-powered. Neither type will remove 'eyes' or bad spots. All electric potato peelers are attachments to mixers: at present, there are none available in this country as a separate family-sized item. They work by spinning the potatoes in a drum which drives them against an abrasive wall and scrapes off the skin.

In the case of water-powered peelers, the potatoes, enclosed in the container with a clamped lid, are rotated against abrasive walls by water power provided by a hose fixed to the tap. Those with weak hands may find it difficult to fix the lid clamp or to push the hose onto the tap. Care must be taken that the force of the water does not disconnect the hose.

2. Some firms specialising in aids (as opposed to retail shops) supply standard swivel peelers fixed to a clamp (Figure 3.12); the peel should not fall to the floor as the peeler is angled to prevent this.

Since the vegetable is peeled by scraping it against the blade of the peeler, this type is particularly helpful to people with the use of only one hand. When trying to decide which to buy, weigh the merits of this peeler against an aid which fixes the vegetable instead of the peeler; the latter might be more versatile (see spike boards, p. 70).

In addition, consider whether you are strong enough to tighten the clamp on the worktop, and remember that you cannot see the area being peeled unless you put the vegetable behind the peeler as you work. Otherwise, the vegetable has to be turned constantly so that you can see which areas to attack next.

3. Those hand-held peelers available in the shops offer a range of both handles and function. Swivel double-edged peelers, suitable for both left and right-handed people, are particularly useful to a household which includes both left and right-handed members. They can also be used to peel towards or away from you. Left-handed peelers are also available for those who prefer them.

Hoop-handled peelers have a double blade and a handle that is generally easier to grip than the standard knife handle (Figure 3.13). The peeling action — pulling towards you — requires little or no wrist movement,

Figure 3.12: Swivel Peeler Fixed to Clamp

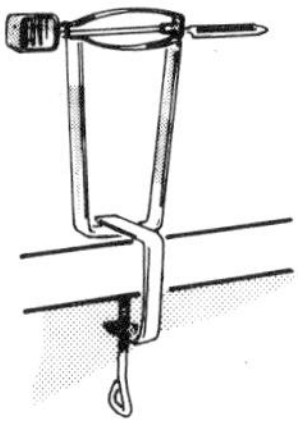

Figure 3.13: Rex Peeler with Loop Handle

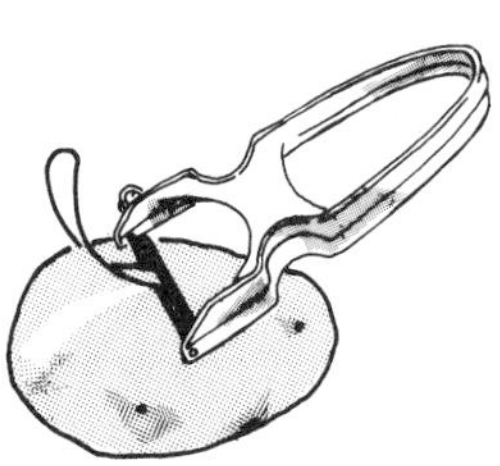

and these peelers are equally easy for left or right-handed people. They also have a hook for removing 'eyes'.

If you have to peel vegetables by hand, remember that peeling a large one is less work than peeling several small ones. This is also true of scrubbed vegetables.

Enlarging Handles

See section on 'Eating' (p. 95).

Spike Boards

Vegetables can be held firm while being peeled if they are impaled on the three or four spikes set upright in a wooden or metal board (Figure 3.14). Spike boards are particularly useful for anyone using only one hand (as long as the hand is kept well away from the spikes).

One make has a rasper attached beside the spikes so that vegetables can be scraped clean instead of being peeled (Figure 3.15). Some people have found the rasper unsatisfactory, and particularly difficult to clean after use; it gets clogged easily, and some pressure must be exerted if the vegetable is to be peeled satisfactorily. The spike section is rather near the rasper but can be obtained as a separate item.

If you have poor sight, the following tips might be helpful: peel potatoes dry to ensure that there is an easily felt difference in texture between the peeled and unpeeled surface; peel downwards from top to bottom while rotating the potato clockwise.

Chopping/Slicing

For chopping with a *knife*, one that has a long blade is generally recommended as it has a straight cutting edge and a substantial handle. Keep it sharp by using an inexpensive knife sharpener which can be mounted on the wall (or brought out as required) so that the blade of the knife can be drawn several times across the groove. One knife sharpener is made with a handle which makes it easy to use, and another has a suction base.

Knives with an 'ergonomic' handle — one that stands at right-angles to

Figure 3.14: Spike Board with Buttering Edge

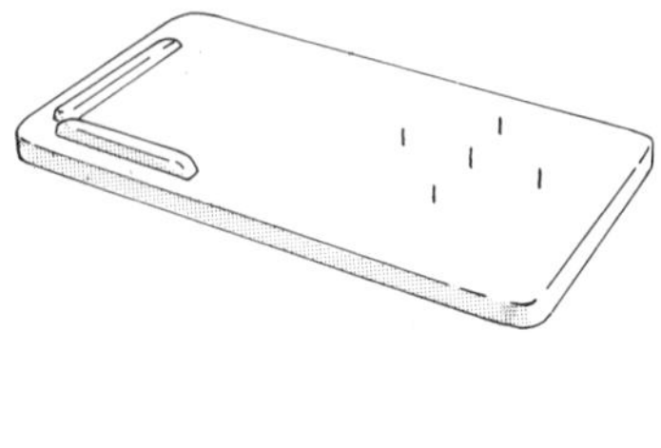

Figure 3.15: Clyde Potato Peeler

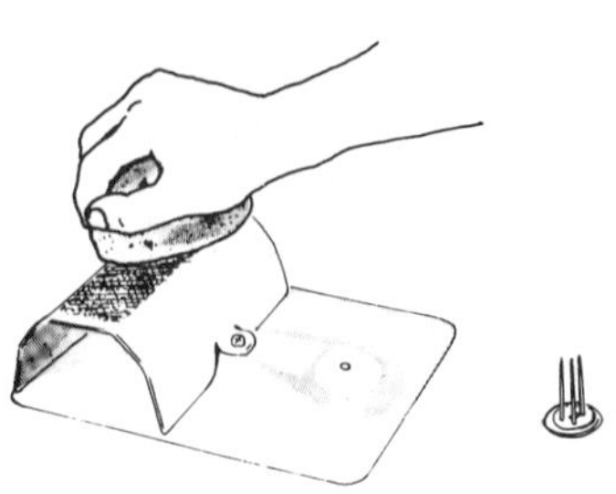

the blade — might be particularly useful to people with weak grip or stiff wrists. These have a long blade similar to a French knife and are available with a serrated or plain edge (Figure 3.16).

Various makes of *autochop* — a spring-loaded knife protected in a canister and worked by sharply pressing down on the knob on top of the canister — are available. Some strength is needed to operate these, but no fine movements are required: they are safe to use, although potentially dangerous to wash as the zigzag blade just shows below the inside of the canister. They require some dexterity and strength to dismantle; try this before buying. Some people find electric knives/carvers useful to cut meat; they might prove heavy for others.

Scissors have innumerable uses in the kitchen but the weight and size of handles may present problems. Many people prefer needlework scissors to the kitchen type as they are lighter, sharper and smaller, and therefore cut more precisely. As well as cutting bacon, parsley and meat, scissors are often indispensable for opening difficult packaging such as polythene wraps on frozen foods, milk cartons and foil-wrapped goods. In addition, visually handicapped people often find them easier to use for cutting than knives. They *must* be kept sharp.

Long or short-bladed scissors of many types can be bought in the shops, with various sizes of finger holes. Also available are 'snips', designed for cutting almost anything from rose stems to thick cardboard; these have spring-loaded handles similar to secateurs, and have the added advantage that you cannot cut yourself on them. Other scissors of various lengths with spring hoop handles have the advantage that the user does not have to put his fingers into the holes; they are available from mail order firms. Some standard scissors are spring loaded which can be helpful.

Other Aids to Chopping. An 'onion stick', which has ten equally spaced prongs about 75 mm (3 in) long set in a plastic handle, can be pushed into a vegetable or fruit to hold it steady while it is sliced between the prongs — a very neat way to slice onions, beetroot or anything similar (Figure 3.17).

Figure 3.16: Ergonomic Knife with Right-angled Grip

Figure 3.17: Onion Stick

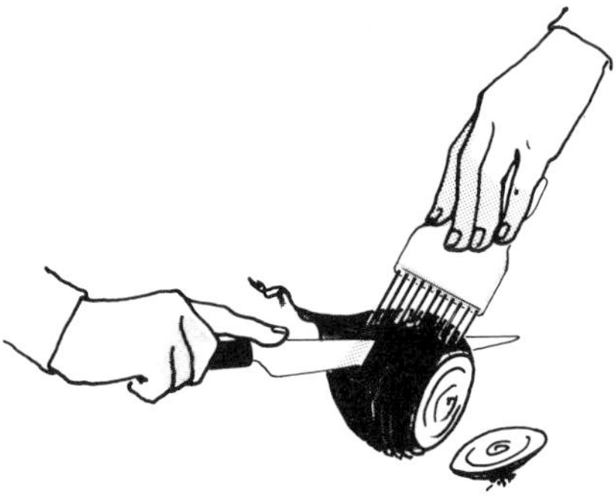

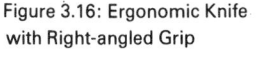

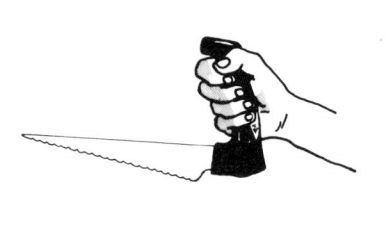

Tomatoes will need a serrated knife to make slicing successful. A large fork can sometimes be used in the same way.

A blender, which can be bought either as part of a mixer or on its own, will chop anything very finely — from vegetables or fruit to bread (for making breadcrumbs) (see Chapter 2, p. 46).

A food processor has a variety of grating and chopping accessories and will slice or grate at great speed. The food will probably have to be cut into small even-sized pieces before putting it through the processor (see Chapter 2, p. 46).

Ideas for Chopping Parsley and Mint

1. Buy ready prepared (dried) herbs, if possible.
2. If fresh, prepare and chop more than you need, pat dry in a cloth and store in the fridge in a polythene bag or yoghurt carton; the chopped leaves will keep for several days.
3. Some people find it easier to place the leaves in a cup or mug and cut them up with scissors.
4. Small mouli-type choppers cut parsley and mint. Chopped parsley or mint can be frozen in blocks in the ice-tray of the fridge to be thawed when needed and, if you have a microwave cooker, herbs can be dried very quickly in it.

Cutting Bread

1. Buy sliced bread.
2. Fix the loaf on a meat carving board (with spikes) or a 'suregrip' spike-board.
3. A sharp carving knife or an electric knife may be easier to use than a breadsaw.
4. A specially designed breadboard with an upstanding slot for the knife and a bar will hold the bread in the right position. This is useful for people with unsteady hands or poor sight (Figure 3.18). (The largest size of loaf may not fit into the frame.)
5. Some people find rotary meat slicers useful for slicing other things but it is doubtful whether their usefulness outweighs their dangers, and they are likely to be expensive.
6. A box has been designed to hold a loaf with a slot for the knife to cut evenly.

Figure 3.18: Combined Bread Board and Knife

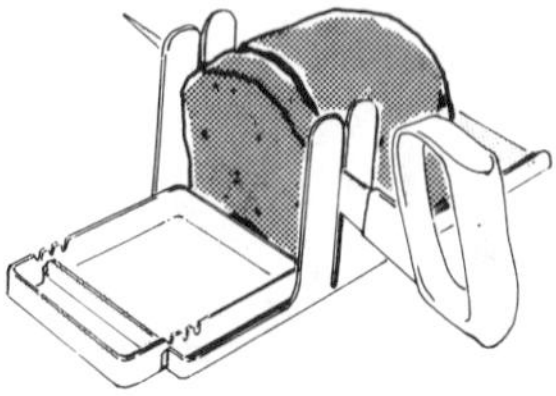

7. The 'Dux' knife has a slicer attachment which holds the blade in the chosen place to cut an even slice. Visually handicapped people find this particularly useful.

Spreading Bread

Plain wooden boards with beading along two sides against which bread can be pushed are useful for one-handed people and possibly for others as well. One-handed people can spread (like peeling a potato) by pulling the knife towards them, supporting the bread on the thumb. The board needs a slip-resistant material underneath to stop it sliding on the worktop surface. Soft margarine is softer than butter when used straight from the fridge.

Ideas for Cutting and Mincing Meat

1. Buy meat already cut if possible. Supermarkets sell some stewing meat ready-cut, and some butchers will trim it as well.
2. Always keep the carving knife very sharp (see also the section on electric knives, p. 47).
3. Various hand-turned mincers, operated by a lever, with either a clamp or suction feet are available. Also, food processors mince meat very quickly, some electric mixers have mincer attachments and there are electrical appliances for shredding and mincing.
4. A butcher, if asked, will mince meat.

Grating

Box-type or pyramid shaped graters with a handle over the top are the most stable — a hand rested on top will hold them steady. A fixture to hold a grater can be bought or made if necessary. Stainless steel and plastic graters are available; the stainless steel ones are much sharper.

Flat graters slide onto a special box to catch the bits as they are grated; these are especially helpful for visually handicapped people. The box needs to sit on a slip-resistant mat or base but is very stable to use. Food processors probably offer the easiest and fastest way to grate and mince food (see Chapter 2, p. 46).

Straining Vegetables

Place the vegetables in a cooking basket (there are different types available; some rigid, some collapsible) or a chip basket within the saucepan so that they automatically drain as they are lifted out. Steamers that fit over pans have the advantage that the pan lid can still be used when cooking, whereas some of the baskets make this impossible. Alternatively, after first placing a damp cloth on the edge of the sink, pull the pan to the edge and tip all the contents into a collander placed in the sink.

Straining lids are not recommended since the pan must be lifted for a long time while the lid is held on.

Pouring

If your hands are shaky, you may find plastic jugs with hinged lids helpful. You need not lift a kettle or jug if you stand the vessel into which you are pouring in the sink, and rest the kettle or jug on a damp cloth on the side of the draining board to tilt it. Use the same principle in other situations — making the vessel from which you are pouring higher than the one which is being filled. A cup of stock being poured into a pan or bowl is steadier if you stand the cup on something that makes it the same height as the bowl, so that all you have to do is to tilt it. Using a funnel is the best way of filling anything with a narrow top; one funnel has a collar to prevent blow-back (see also p. 101).

Peeling Fruit

The aids available for peeling vegetables can also be used to peel some fruit, though there are some extra hints worth knowing.

1. Oranges are easier to peel if they are first brought to the boil in a pan of water, and then put into cold water.
2. Tomatoes should be placed in boiling water for a few seconds before being peeled or held on a fork in a gas flame until the skin splits.
3. When making a fruit salad, it is sometimes easier to slice a whole orange across the segments rather than pull the segments apart with the fingers. A curved 'slicing knife' (available from household stores) makes thin slicing easier.
4. Cut unpeeled oranges into about eight segments, starting by cutting them in half across; the pieces are easy to hold while biting into the flesh of the fruit.
5. Halve an orange and eat it with a spoon, like grapefruit.

Apples. To save peeling cooking apples, remove the stalks, wash and quarter them straight into a pan with very little water. The contents of the pan can then be put through a sieve or mouli-mill when cooked. For other methods of peeling, see p. 68.

Stoning Fruit. Most people cook fruit with the stones in. However, those who prefer their fruit 'stoned' should remember that gadgets for removing stones from cherries and plums are as difficult to operate as garden secateurs. 'Stoners' are available from ordinary household stores.

Making Cakes and Pastry

Weighing/Sieving

Weighing.
1. One of the most important factors to consider when choosing scales is the stability of the pan.

2. Wall scales naturally give greater stability than free-standing ones, and the pan folds away when not in use.
3. Those with poor sight will probably find scales with weights easier to use than spring balance ones. If spring balance scales are preferred, however, choose those which have as large a division between the marks as possible for accurate weighing; in addition, scales with braille markings on them are available.

Some scales make it easy to see the small weights often needed when cooking; the weights are shown on a clock face — the equivalent of 1 to 3 o'clock showing the large scale divisions (0 to 4450g; 0 to 16oz), while from 3 to 12 o'clock shows (0.3 to 4.5kg; 1 to 10lb) in less detail. Easy types of scales include a jug type with a handle and spout, and those with a dial which can be returned to zero so that other ingredients can be added.

Some find a measure easier to manage than scales. A measure is marked for many kinds of dry ingredients and is less expensive than scales; however, some are less accurate and not very easy to see.

Many basic recipes can be made using just a yoghurt pot as a convenient measure of volume (see Chapter 7).

Sieving. A bulldog clip or clothes peg will fix a strainer to the side of the bowl to keep it steady.

Mixing/Beating

A lot of effort will be saved if the bowl is fixed before mixing starts; for one-handed people, this is an obvious necessity. There are various ways of doing this.

1. Obtain a Dycem mat or sheet (see p. 64).
2. Stand the bowl on a damp dishcloth or plastic foam sheeting.
3. Sit down and mix with the bowl on your lap.
4. Put the bowl in the sink — especially if your arms are painful or weak and you work more easily at a lower level, also if you are shaky or if you have a visual handicap — so that you need not worry about the mess if something spills.
5. 'Bowl holders', that is, holes the size of standard bowls, can be made in a pull-out worktop and the efficiency of these can be improved still further if a foam strip is stuck around the rims of the holes. A unit with the same type of holes that can stand or a work top is also available.
6. Use a rubber bowl holder on a suction base with a dip in the top to hold the bowl.
7. Suction pads of various kinds can be useful. The Stayput Pad is a non-slip pad 10cm in diameter which is placed on a smooth surface. The object to be secured can be pressed lightly on the pad and rotated to form an effective seal. By rotating in the opposite direction the seal can be easily broken. Alternatively, some people find that double suction cups fix a bowl

successfully — or a suction soap holder, obtainable from chemists' shops and hardware stores, can be used. Suction pads of this kind raise the base of the bowl above the work surface and might cause the bowl to wobble about while the mixture is being stirred; the other ways suggested to keep it steady are possibly better.

Types of Mixing Bowl

Plastic. Polythene bowls are inclined to be too light to be stable, and, as they scratch easily, are not very hygienic. However, melamine bowls are thicker, heavier, and are deep and stable. Some have a pouring lip. Scratching will impair the shiny surface but not so badly as the less rigid plastic. Plastic bowls are the only ones that are not noisy to use.

Stainless Steel. This type is light, hygienic and unbreakable.

Enamel. These bowls are attractive and have the same properties as steel, except that they chip easily if dropped or knocked; they are likely to be cheaper than steel.

Glass. These are fairly heavy to lift and easily broken; but they look, and are, hygienic. However, they are almost impossible to see if you have a visual handicap, and should be avoided at all costs.

Earthenware. This type of bowl is stable, although comparatively heavy and easily broken or chipped. It is hygienic while it remains uncracked.

Points about Mixing

Food preparation machines make it possible to use many recipes that might otherwise be difficult or impossible. The many types on the market range from the hand-held to the full-sized mixer with its own bowl (which, however, can be heavy to move). Some of the smaller sized mixers (hand-held or with their own bowl and stand) are reasonably light, although the beaters may be difficult to release. Food processors need to be carefully chosen to ensure that they suit the purchaser's particular abilities; they are not very light, some are difficult to dismantle, they do not mix creamed mixtures as well as a conventional mixer and it is easy to over-process when using one, although practice and experience will overcome this. If possible, to save lifting, keep the mixer where it can be pushed to the back of the work surface after use.

Hand-held mixers have been used successfully by people with very weak hands. They will not mix heavy doughs but some have alternative 'heads' and can be used for chopping as well as mixing. Try the controls and practise dismantling the mixer in the shop before you buy.

Food processors and mixers are discussed in detail in Chapter 2 (see p. 46).

Trying to mix a stiff mixture with a large spoon can be a great strain on wrists and hands; the task will be eased if the ingredients are first broken up with a pastry blender or knife.

Warming the sugar before adding the fat for creaming eases mixing, as does warming the mixing bowl beforehand as long as it does not get too hot.

One-stage cake making is the easiest method; special soft 'tub' margarines make this even easier.

Someone who is one-handed and finds it difficult to scrape the spoon clean, should try using a wire mixer (pastry blender or a strong wire whisk) which can be knocked clean on the side of the bowl, or a flat spatula which can be scraped clean on the side. Some very pliable spatulas and scrapers are available.

Points about Beating and Whisking

Several non-electric whisks are suitable for one-handed use — for example, the wire coil-spring type (Figure 3.19), or those that work by a pressure-release spiral action (Figure 3.20). It is possible to have a stand made so that a rotary whisk can be used with one hand.

Blenders can be bought as a unit or with a mixer. Some also have grinding attachments (see Chapter 2, p. 46).

Electric mixers have whisk attachments and attachments for mincing are also available. Some hand-held electric whisks are also extremely useful for lighter mixtures.

Mixing Pastry

A wire pastry blender, ideal for anyone who is one-handed, is also generally useful as it keeps the pastry cool while mixing. It can also be used for mixing cakes and is easy to clean.

A roller with a central spindle is less tiring on the wrists. Use the roller to lift pastry on to pies (just roll the pastry on to it, and then unroll across the baking dish). If you are visually handicapped, the following method will

Figure 3.19: Wire Whisk (Ritter Quirl)

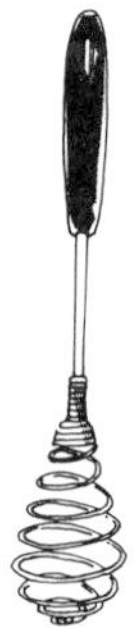

Figure 3.20: Spring-loaded Beater

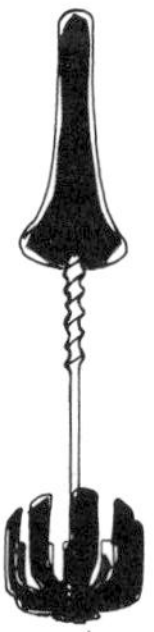

help you to roll out the pastry evenly. Obtain two flat sticks (about 35 × 2.5 × 0.6 cm; 14 × 1 × ¼in) from a wood merchant. Lightly flour the sticks, and lay them on either side of the lump of pastry so that each end of the rolling pin gradually comes to rest on them as the pastry is rolled out to 0.6 cm (¼in) thick all over. The sticks do not slip if you roll straight back and forward only. Plastic rulers could be used for thinner pastry. Pastry cutters with hoop handles may be easier to hold.

Frozen pastry (whether puff, flaky or short) is excellent in quality and saves effort which may be better used elsewhere. Making a large quantity yourself and freezing it for later use is also time-saving.

Greasing Baking Tins. Use a pastry brush and a little softened margarine, cooking fat or oil to grease a tin. Non-stick baking tins are comparatively expensive but are a sound investment. Another alternative is to line cake tins with a piece of greaseproof or baking paper — this is useful even if you have non-stick tins.

Putting Mixture into Tins. Stabilise the tins on a damp cloth. Dip the spoon in hot water as you work — this makes the mixture drop more easily. An ice-cream scoop will do the job neatly and can be operated with only one hand.

Breaking/Separating Eggs.

Breaking Eggs. It is possible to break an egg with one hand. Crack the egg in the normal way on the side of the bowl, then pull the egg apart — with the thumb and first two fingers holding one half and the ring and and little finger holding the other.

If you drop the egg into the bowl from about 30 cm (12 in) above it, the egg will break in half and you can hook out the two halves of shell with your thumb. (Opinions vary as to how successful this method is.) If you find this a difficult job, ask a friend to break an egg or two to store in the fridge in plastic cartons for future use.

If some of the shell falls into the egg when it is broken, an easy way to remove it is to use another piece of shell as a scoop. Some people prefer to use a spoon.

Left-over egg yolk will keep for a few days in the refrigerator if covered with a layer of cold water in a covered container.

Separating Eggs. Egg separators do the job neatly; they are like a deep spoon with holes in the side and sit over a cup like a tea strainer. These are especially useful for people with visual handicap.

Alternatively, break the egg onto a saucer, cover the yolk with an egg cup and hold it there while you tip off the white.

Cooking

Using the Cooker Hob

Not everyone who becomes disabled can afford to buy a new cooker even if the old one has features that are difficult to use. A wheelchair user faced with a free-standing cooker cannot see into the pans. One way around this is to have a 'non-steam' mirror fixed at an angle above the hob; or a mirror on a stick might be more versatile.

A lot of electric cookers have the controls situated at the back of the hob. Some people with stiff shoulders find that they can turn on the cooker without help if they use a stick with a 'thimble' on one end that fits the knobs. Motoring shops sell sticks with suction pads on one or both ends which will do this job.

In some kitchens, it might be possible to clear a space beside the cooker so that the cook can reach the controls from there.

Points about Stirring

1. Work at the right height to save aching arms and back.
2. Make sure the pan is stable first.
3. 'Balloon' whisks are often easier to use than spoons to push around the pan, and particularly useful in substances inclined to 'lump'. (If you are using a non-stick pan, invest in a wooden or plastic whisk which does not scratch.)
4. Look at the different stirring spoons available — long and short handles, fat or thin, large or small bowls to the spoon and an infinite variety of different shapes, wooden or plastic. Spoons with a hole in the middle of the bowl help to prevent lumps in a mixture.
5. Remember that it is easier to stir when the pan is not full, and that long-handled spoons are safest for those with loss of sensation.

Stabilising Pans on the Hob

1. Panguards — small fences that can be fitted round the hob — are designed to stop children pulling pans off the stove, but can be used to push the pans against while stirring. However, they do make it impossible for the pans to be slid across from hob to worktop because the pan must be lifted over the top of the guard. This could be dangerous if the pan base catches on the edge of the guard.
2. One or two pans full of water placed at the back of the stove can be used as stabilisers if, while stirring, the pan in front is swung round so that its handle rests against the one at the back.
3. Pan handle holders are available to attach to the cooker hob.
4. Heavy bottomed pans are more stable than light ones, but are often painfully heavy to lift, even when empty.
5. Visually handicapped people usually feel safest using the back, rather than the front rings, of a hob.

Choosing Cooking Utensils

The variety of cooking utensils is such that everyone should be able to find pans to suit them. Many of us tend to keep old favourites far too long, saddling ourselves with awkward pans which are very difficult to clean, often too heavy or too light, perhaps with uncomfortable or even unsafe handles. It is false economy to keep such pans and it is worth spending time in a good household or department store assessing what best suits your individual needs.

No longer is it necessary to buy 'matching sets' of which possibly only one or two get regular use. A small family is much better served with two or three saucepans all the same size, plus one small frying/omelette pan. Handle the pans before buying to make sure they are well-balanced and comfortable to hold. Those with short, chunky handles and large saucepan knobs are easiest to use. Pans with two handles may be easier to lift than those with one, although they may make straining difficult (see 'Straining', p. 73). Do not be tempted by very cheap, light pans which will soon buckle and burn. A very heavy pan is not essential either. Rather, go for a middle-range, good quality pan, of which there are many, most of which are suitable for gas and electric cookers including ceramic hobs.

Above all, look for a range with non-stick linings which are easy to clean and save so much effort. These need not be expensive and replacing the pan when the surface wears out is more practical than struggling to clean one with a 'sticky' patch.

Specialised Utensils

In addition to conventional saucepans, one or two other popular utensils are particularly useful.

Pressure Cookers. Modern pressure cookers are smaller and lighter than their forebears and their larger handles make them easier to move. But, with food inside, they can still be too heavy and some people may find the lids awkward to fix. They are so economical and take such a short time to cook either the tougher cuts of meat or even a complete meal, that they are well worth consideration.

No longer do they emit clouds of steam or piercing whistles, so they need not frighten anyone. New models do not require elaborate weights, are much quieter in operation, and have simple controls and indicators built into their lids.

Steamers. Steamers also save energy by cooking several types of food one above the other on the same ring, but as the steam in these is not under pressure, cooking in this way takes considerably longer. The simplest steamers are lightweight aluminium or bamboo (Chinese) containers which fit over existing saucepans. The manufacturers of the various steam cookers, dry cookers and waterless cookers on the market make spectacular claims. It is always wise to look into these claims thoroughly before deciding if one is right for you. Better still, if one is recommended by a friend, ask if you can borrow it first to try it at home.

Steaming is used a lot in Chinese cooking, which is not only popular, but nutritionally good, and quick and easy to do (see below).

Woks. These Chinese-style utensils are large, round, metal cooking pots, with a rounded base. Deeper than frying pans, but wider and shallower than most saucepans, they usually have two handles which some disabled cooks prefer. Some models made specially for the Western market have non-stick linings and a stabilising ring to stand them on. They can be used for several different cooking operations — boiling, simmering, deep frying and shallow frying.

Frying

Frying carries the highest fire risk in cooking — especially deep fat frying. The following is a blueprint for successful deep frying.

1. For peace of mind, invest in a thermostatically controlled electric deep fryer, which takes care of all the safety factors automatically (see p. 39). One gas hotplate has a thermostatically controlled burner for safe frying. It senses the temperature of the fat in the pan and reduces the flame when the correct temperature is reached.
2. Use a deep, straight-sided pan. A large saucepan is often better than a so-called 'chip pan' because it is deeper and allows room for the frying medium to bubble up without spilling over. Make sure the pan is wide enough to cover the source of heat.
3. Use a good quality frying oil rather than a hard fat. Not only is this better nutritionally, but oil has a higher 'flash point' which means it is not so likely to burst spontaneously into flames.
4. Fill the pan no more than one-third full of oil. It should not be more than two-thirds full when the food has been added, again allowing room for the hot fat to bubble up safely.
5. Heat the fat gently until the required temperature has been reached. For chips, it should be hot enough to brown a small cube of bread in one minute. Better still, invest in a frying thermometer and use that. For chips, use a temperature of 190°C (380°F). Other larger items of food need correspondingly lower temperatures, between 170°C (340°F) and 185°C (360°F).
6. *Never* cover the pan while the oil is heating nor during cooking.
7. Never leave the pan unattended during heating or cooking. If the door bell or telephone rings, *turn off the heat* before answering it.
8. When frying is finished, turn off the heat, put the lid on the pan and leave it where it is until it is cold. Then strain it if necessary and return it to

the cleaned pan or other suitable container, covered, until required again.

9. Replace frying oil when it is discoloured or if it has become overheated.

10. If these rules are followed, frying is perfectly safe. But always keep ready either a large metal baking tray, a fire blanket or a wrung-out damp tea towel. If the worst happens and the fat pan should catch fire, *do not attempt to move it*, but turn off the heat at once, and cover the flames with the tray, blanket or tea towel. The flames will be extinguished almost at once, but leave everything where it is until the pan is quite cold.

Many recipes specify that the food should be fried or grilled; the same result can often be achieved if it is baked in the oven. Also, cooking oven chips avoids the hazards involved in deep fat frying and the problems of peeling and cutting potatoes.

Boiling Eggs

Those who find it difficult to take the eggs out of the pan might try boiling them in a vegetable cooking basket or in an egg holder on a central handle which stands in the pan and holds up to four eggs.

Using the Oven

Cookers are discussed in detail in Chapter 2.

Gas Lighters. If you have to light your own oven and have difficulty in reaching the burners, consider the following:

fasten a taper on a stick (or perhaps a bamboo cane) with a rubber band (not a wax taper or the drips will block the gas burner);

sit down to light it;

use long 'gift shop' matches;

look for a gas lighter with a long nozzle;

if you are visually handicapped, look for a lighter which emits a continuous stream of sparks, each spark being accompanied by a click.

Points about Baking

Small baking tins, pie dishes and casseroles are easier to lift when placed on a baking tray or in a shallow roasting or swiss-roll pan. The tray also catches any spills. If using a baking sheet, make sure that you can keep it level as you lift, or the casserole is likely to slide off the back. Casseroles with one handle (pottery ones with the handle built in) have been recommended by one-handed people and those who have to work one-handed because they have to steady themselves with the other hand. Getting cakes out of the tin and washing up afterwards are made easier if non-stick cake tins are used. Cake tins with removable bases are comparatively easy to use, and the cake can be left on the base for cutting and serving.

Points about Roasting

Before putting the tin into the oven, check that it is not too heavy to lift with the joint inside it. Alternatively, wrap the meat in foil and place it directly on a shelf with a roasting pan underneath to collect the drips (foil used inside out reduces reflection of heat in an oven).

To save mess, cover the meat tin with foil, or use a covered dish or roasting bag; if you wrap the meat in foil, be careful of hot liquid when you unwrap it.

Enamel roasting tins with lids, which usually have a handle at each end, may be easier to lift than plain tins.

Remember that food cooked in a covered tin needs no basting (or you can cover the tin with foil). If you want to baste, consider using a basting syringe rather than a spoon. Fat splashing is cut down if you put the roast in a tin that is only just large enough to accommodate it.

Getting Dishes Out of the Oven

Make sure you are adequately protected from the heat before you start. A trolley with a gently sloping ramp added, which helps to avoid lifting, is especially useful to the one-handed housewife. The ramp can be hinged to one shelf of a wooden trolley with hooks to rest on the edge of the oven rack (Figure 3.21). (This would have to be specially made — at the moment there are no ready-made trolleys with ramps.) REMAP (Rehabilitation Engineering Movement Advisory Panel) designs and makes special items to meet individual needs. If you need a 'one-off' piece of kitchen equipment, contact the local authority's social services department or the area health authority, both of which work closely with REMAP.

Figure 3.21: Trolley with Sloping Ramp

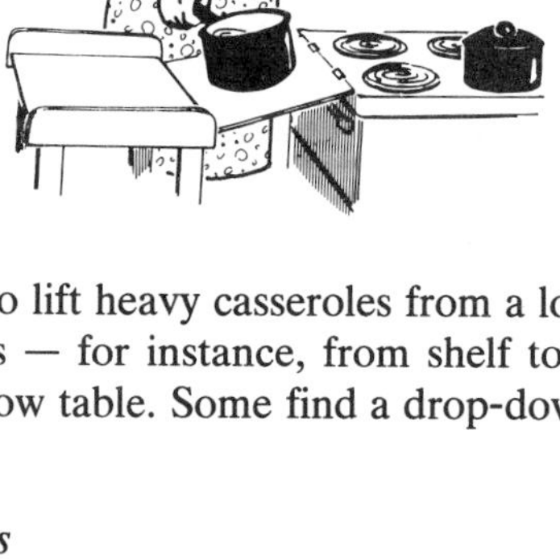

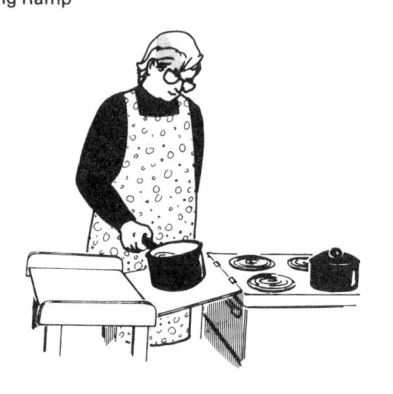

If you find it difficult to lift heavy casseroles from a low oven to a work top, try doing it in stages — for instance, from shelf to a steady stool or chair seat, from stool to low table. Some find a drop-down oven door useful as a first stage.

Points about Oven Gloves

1. The kind made in a strip with a mitt at each end protect the arms to

some extent, but may, however, be too thick for some people to feel what they are doing. It is possible to extend the depth of the glove by sewing pieces of oven cloth to the top edges of the mitts.

2. Oven gloves (separate for each hand, with thumbs) are available in different lengths, the longest reaching to just below the elbow.

3. If you use an ordinary cloth, make sure it is thick enough to be really heat-proof, but at the same time not so thick that it is resistant to bending round your hands and the object. The best type to use is one that is thick enough when single. It should be big enough to cover each hand and go round your largest casserole.

4. Make sure the oven gloves or cloth are dry when used — a damp cloth will make steam and scald your hands while the hot dish is being carried.

5. Wheelchair users removing hot casseroles from oven to lap usually have their own ideas for protection from heat. One possibility is to have a wooden (slip-resistant) chopping board on your lap; a quilted apron is also useful.

If you have someone else at home and cannot reach some part of the cooker (usually the grill or oven), ask them to put the meal in the oven in the morning, so that you can turn it on at the right time.

Most electric and gas ovens have an automatic time switch that turns the oven on and off at the times set; also some gas ovens have 'slow' settings which allow the food to be cooked for long periods (6 to 10 hours); this is a good way to cook cheap cuts of meat. See also 'Slow cookers', p. 39.

Using the Refrigerator

A medium-sized refrigerator is as much a part of the kitchen as the cooker, so make sure it is included in your normal routine. It may be easier to use and keep tidy if it is raised to a convenient height on a sturdy plinth.

Get into the habit of unpacking perishable shopping and putting it straight into the refrigerator, keeping an eye on its contents, using it to keep food fresh and clean, and using food before it is stale. Remember — a fridge keeps perishable food fresh for longer, but it does not prolong its life indefinitely.

Points about Using a Refrigerator

1. When choosing a new model, think about getting one which defrosts itself automatically. It may cost a little more, but will save a lot of trouble.

2. If using a model which needs manual defrosting, try to do it regularly and fairly frequently, then there will not be a big build-up of ice to remove.

3. Once the ice round the evaporator has melted, leave the water in the tray beneath until a sheet of ice has formed on the top. It will then be easier to carry the tray to the sink to empty it, without spillage. Defrosting more often means less water. Each manufacturer's instruction leaflet gives full instructions for carrying out this simple operation.

4. When putting new purchases in the fridge, transfer foods from paper bags and wraps to clean plastic bags to keep them from drying out. Ordinary lightweight plastic bags saved from shopping are quite suitable for this short-term storage.
5. Do not leave the door open longer than necessary when in use, as the warm air entering the cabinet raises the temperature (causing frost to form more quickly) and increases the running costs.
6. Wipe milk bottles before putting away to save marks on the plastic shelves. Pour milk from cartons into a lidded jug or measure.
7. Save and wash plastic cartons, preferably with lids, such as margarine and yoghurt pots, and use for keeping small quantities of left-over vegetables, rice and sauces in the fridge until the next day.
8. Left-over cold cooked meat is most easily stored on a plate, putting the whole thing inside a large, clean, plastic bag.
9. Make full use of the vegetable drawer and specially designed fittings on the door, but do not worry about special places for various foods. They may all be placed on any shelf.
10. Keep a supply of ice-cubes always to hand in a plastic box in the evaporator.
11. Prepare food ahead and leave ready to cook the next day.
12. Use to hasten the setting of jellies and other cold sweets.

Using the Freezer

Although freezers are comparatively new to our kitchens, many consider they are essential for people with any kind of disability, for their sheer convenience and for the insurance they offer against 'off days'. An upright front-opening model is much easier to use (see Chapter 2, p. 50).

Points about Using a Freezer

1. Some long-established habits of shopping and budgeting may have to be revised at first, but once a new routine is established, a freezer can save endless worry over shopping, catering and entertaining.
2. Buy and follow a good freezer instruction book. After about six months, the simple rules will become second nature. Remember that everything can be frozen — some foods are more successful than others, and some frozen foods appeal more to one person than another.
3. Although many specialised packing materials are available, the only really necessary ones are plastic boxes, plastic bags and adhesive labels. For freezer storage, it is essential to use the proper, heavier gauge plastic bags sold for the purpose and obtainable from most department stores, large grocers, chemists, or by mail order. But plastic lidded cartons can also be saved and used to hold small quantities of food in the freezer.
4. Labelling is also essential to help locate food easily, as well as to identify it. Try also to keep similar kinds of food together — on separate shelves, in cardboard boxes or in net bags.

5. Cling film is a very useful wrapping material for storing food in both fridge and freezer, but it can be tricky to handle. Special boxes and wall-mounted holders with serrated edges are available but, if it is difficult to handle these, try the following method: (1) place the food to be wrapped on a heavy chopping board and drop the roll of cling film behind it. Now both hands are free; (2) pull the film over the food, tuck it underneath and roll the food up, covering it with several thicknesses of film; (3) cut the film with the tip of a pointed knife and press it closely to the food, excluding as much air as possible. Cling film is self-adhesive, so does not need any other fastening, but if the food is to be frozen, put the whole thing into a labelled plastic bag.
6. Some kinds of protective gloves are useful when handling frozen foods, especially by those with delicate skin. Loose cotton gloves are probably best.
7. Defrost the freezer regularly and fairly frequently, to make this job as simple as possible. A plan for defrosting is given on p. 51 in Chapter 2, or follow the manufacturer's instructions.
8. Give the outside of both the freezer and the fridge a quick wipe over about once a week to remove fingermarks and splashes. Just use clean detergent suds before you start washing up to save making it a separate job.

Using the Sink

Turning the sink taps on and off can be difficult. Taps come in many shapes and sizes and are often difficult to grasp. Unless you have electronic automatic taps, a tap with a lever handle is probably the easiest to turn; however, it is not always convenient to have existing taps exchanged for lever taps.

The following might be acceptable alternatives:

1. a lever tap handle (such as the Shavrin), easily fitted to any kind of tap, replaces the top half of the tap, and can be obtained in different colours for hot and cold;
2. various tap-turning aids which fit over the existing tap. The handles are available in different lengths, and vary in design to suit the different types of existing knobs.

Lifting pans and kettles for filling can be avoided if a short hose is fitted on the tap. A swivel tap can be useful in a similar way. See also Chapter 1, p. 11, for points to consider when choosing taps.

Sinks for Wheelchair Users

A sink that is only 5 in deep (see also Chapter 1, p. 10) enables a wheelchair user to wheel right up to the sink with the knees underneath it; it can also benefit those with back pain or limited arm movement who find it difficult to lift from the bottom of a deep sink to the draining board (Figure 3.22). If you have this type, make sure that the underside of the sink is insulated to prevent your knees getting burnt. Remember, however, that water splashes more easily out of a shallow sink. A sink placed across a corner provides the washer-up with two adjacent work surfaces and also, if unsteady, with a feeling of security. This is particularly useful for wheelchair users, but it is largely a matter of personal preference.

Figure 3.22: Shallow Sink with Lever Taps

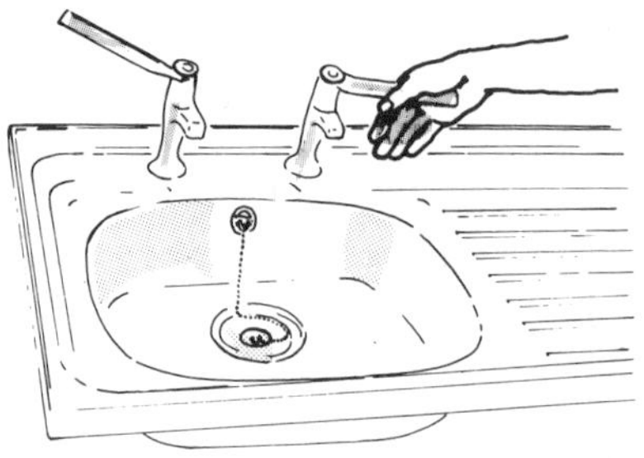

Washing Up

The numerous dishwashers on the market, of various sizes (from floor-standing to small counter-top sized models) and capacities, are considered indispensable by those who own them. They are particularly useful for anyone who has a large family, who entertains often or who has a skin problem which is exacerbated by hot water or detergents. Someone who is inclined to be clumsy may also find that they decrease the number of breakages (see also Chapter 2, p. 52).

Saving Work When Washing Up

1. Use as few utensils as possible, for instance, oven-to-table ware. Cook several items in one saucepan, such as potatoes and another vegetable. There are 'all-in-one' steamers available as an alternative.
2. Use non-stick pans where possible; line the base of baking tins and grill pans with foil before use; rinse or soak dishes as soon as they are used; use really hot water (but not if you have a skin problem).
3. In addition, leave the things to drain instead of drying — even cutlery (there are very good cutlery drainers on the market). If you are visually handicapped, tall items should always be placed at the back of the draining board, that is, close to the wall. A coloured mat (plastic) on the board will make stainless steel cutlery show up against a stainless steel draining board. If you must dry up, sit down to do it. To wring out the dishcloth, put it round the tap and twist the two ends together.
4. For one-handed people, a mop or brush on a suction pad can be fixed

to the side or bottom of the sink, which is also useful for scrubbing vegetables. Otherwise suction cups will hold plates while they are being washed and dried. Some people find it easier to dry up on their lap.

5. Tea cloth holders near the sink are easier to use than a towel rail (particularly those with two opposite brushes which do not have the same tendency to trap the fingers as the rubber ones). The pull-out type of rail, located beside the sink, is preferred by some, while others find it awkward.

Mobility Around the Kitchen

Reaching and Bending

Storing things in the kitchen involves a great deal of reaching and bending (see Chapter 1, p. 14-16). Although it may *not* be possible to alter the present heights or depths of the cupboards and shelves, it may be possible to rearrange the stores and perhaps add various storage aids so that the things that are used most are at a convenient height. As far as china and cutlery are concerned, for example, many housewives store 'one or two of everything' where they can be easily reached and handled.

If cupboards and refrigerator are too low, they can be put on blocks or plinths. If castors are added on the bottom of the plinth, the cupboard or fridge can be both easily reached and pulled out for cleaning. In this case, make sure that they can be firmly fixed or hooked, so that they cannot move on their own. Special rigid stands on castors are available from most large stores to hold heavy appliances like cookers. A fridge freezer with a fridge on the top half might be useful (see Chapter 2, p. 51).

Anyone who is shaky and has to reach down to a low cupboard, should do so from a sitting position. Apart from actual storage, heights of tea towel holders and rubbish bins, for instance, may have to be adjusted. Using the space on the backs of cupboard doors for racks, fixtures and shelves can save more space in a small kitchen than appears at first sight.

A long-handled dustpan can be used to collect items in the bottom of the fridge, so that these can then be lifted to table level and deposited. This idea could perhaps also be used with small items in a low cupboard or to help feed pet animals. This type of dustpan can also be used to scoop up the frost or water from the bottom of a chest freezer when it is being defrosted and cleaned.

Plugs and Sockets

If electric socket outlets (see also Chapter 1, p. 18) are not set on the wall at a height you can reach, get them moved by a qualified electrician. Otherwise, a unit to convert a low socket to a higher one or *vice versa* can be fitted. Another useful gadget is a notched plug holder which holds the plugs at a reachable height ready to be used when required.

Several plugs have grab-handles, either as part of the plug or designed to be attached to it, so that the plug can more easily be pulled out of the socket.

Plugs and sockets are available in bright colours, while braille or large print labels can be bought to stick on the plugs so that, for example, the refrigerator is not unplugged by mistake.

Cleaning up Spills

Messy floors are depressing and can be dangerous. Spilt liquids can make even slip-resistant floors slippery. Anyone who cannot bend to reach spills and any other mess could use:

1. a 'Flexiflow' mop — on a long and bendy handle for getting into corners;
2. a 'Flexiflow' duster — which is the same as the Flexiflow mop but with a shorter handle (both with washable, removable nylon head);
3. a long-handled dustpan and brush. Some are designed so that the brush handle fits into the pan handle when not in use. Others have lids that close automatically when lifted from the floor;
4. some housewives use a 'pick-up-stick' with a cloth in it to wipe the floor (see 'Picking Things Up' below);
5. a housewife who is steady on her feet but can hardly reach with her arms could push a floorcloth round with her feet.

A visually handicapped person cleaning a floor must be very methodical, using the tile line as a marker or perhaps leaving a cloth as a double check on how much has been cleaned. Patterned flooring should be avoided as this limits visibility.

Picking Things Up

Some people who find this a problem use a rod with a hook on the end — some keep several around the house in strategic places. These rods are easy to make out of a length of bamboo or dowelling rod, and are especially useful if articles are stored in containers with hookable handles — for example, bottles and jars in a milk bottle holder.

One aid, used most often to help with dressing, is made from a wooden coat hanger with the hook removed; a small hook is screwed into one end and a rubber 'thimble' over the other end. This has other uses too, especially for anyone who finds a longer rod difficult to manipulate.

Pick-up Sticks

Also known as 'Helping Hands' and 'Reachers', pick-up sticks come in various designs but are basically a rod with a grabbing device at one end and a mechanism for operating it on the other — this being usually either a trigger or a pair of sprung levers which are pulled together in action (see Figure 3.23). Lazy Tongs, similar to extending scissors, are convenient to

Figure 3.23: Easy Reacher Reaching Aid

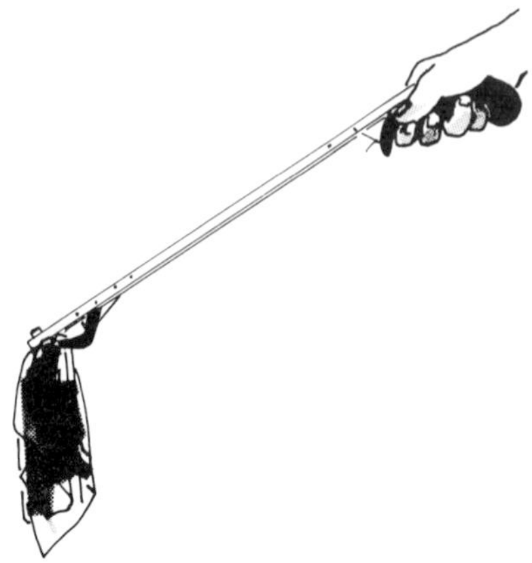

carry around but are limited in what they can pick up and lift, being very small and light.

When choosing a pick-up stick, be sure to try it first and consider:

1. its weight; some are heavy even without a load;
2. the maximum width of the 'jaws', which varies considerably;
3. whether or not the operating mechanism suits the particular ability of your hands;
4. whether it might be sensible to have more than one type varying in weight and height depending on the circumstance in which you might need one;
5. whether a folding reacher would be useful both at home and to take with you when away from home.

People with shaky hands may find lifting a storage jar easier if they remove the lid first so that they can hold the rim of the jar.

Carrying Things

Before reviewing the various types of trolleys and trays that can help to transport items to, from and around the kitchen, consider the various ways of reducing: (1) the need to carry things around in the first place, and (2) the distance they have to be carried. Also, and most important, consider the safety aspect of lifting, for instance, pans, kettles and casseroles, especially when they are hot.

Some useful ideas are:

1. to install a hatchway (as wide as practicable) between the kitchen and dining room (the hatch should have a shelf on each side so that dishes can be moved across easily);
2. to eat in the kitchen;

3. to make sure that the cooker hob, sink rim and adjacent worktops are all at one level so that pots and pans can be dragged to and fro without lifting (see Chapter 1, p. 12);

4. to keep some tea/coffee and a kettle and cup in the living room or bedroom, or wherever refreshment is usually taken, so that a drink can be made on the spot. Some people fill a thermos flask and leave it where it will be needed.

Safety

Plan what you are going to lift and where to, so that the surfaces are clear beforehand; also make sure you can manage the weight of the item before you move it, for instance, a heavy joint of meat (which will also be sitting in hot fat) that has to be lifted from oven to worktop. Remember that the weight of pans and casseroles is mainly affected by the amount of food or liquid in them. Cooking in small amounts lessens the weight and makes spillage less likely.

Trolleys

Trolleys are invaluable (as long as different floor levels do not have to be negotiated). Even then, if the difference is not great, a ramp may be the answer. Trolleys vary in size and weight; some are heavy enough to support the person pushing them while others are light enough to be pushed with a touch (even with the end of a walking stick).

Walking support trolleys include wooden ones of various dimensions with two melamine-covered shelves. The pushing handle is a bar on one end, and the castor wheels are larger than those on some standard trolleys (Figure 3.24). Within this range, there are two alternative heights and two sets of dimensions for either; the smallest has 40 cm (16 in) square trays.

Figure 3.24: Etwall Trolley

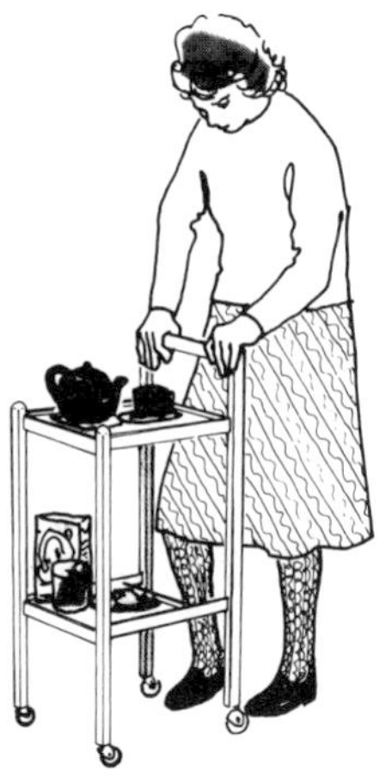

Others of similar design are available, not all with alternative dimensions. Pay particular attention to the castors to see that they are sufficiently large and strong since the castors normally fail before the rest of the trolley. It is worth considering the firmness of the frame since loosening of a frame which cannot be tightened is another cause of trolley failure.

Another type of trolley is made of steel and can be bought with alternative pushing handles – a pushing bar, walking stick type handles or arm support troughs — which are interchangeable on the basic trolley frame. Walking trolleys do not usually have brakes, but the body weight inhibits fast movement. Other walking supports include walking aids designed to take a basket or tray (Figure 3.25). These are particularly useful for shopping, especially those with brakes (Figure 3.26). Walking aids not so designed might topple over if the bag is too full.

Trays

One-handed Trays

Anyone who has only one hand (or who is rendered one-handed, or no-handed, when using a walking aid) will obviously find a standard tea-tray useless, as will a visually handicapped person who needs one hand for guidance. However, various types of trays are designed for one-handed use; either they have a rigid hoop handle over the top — like a basket (Figure 3.27) — or are suspended from a small handgrip above, so that the tray swings (Figure 3.28). This attribute is supposed to prevent spillage of the items carried, by centrifugal force. Some one-handed trays also have a slip-resistant surface (Figure 3.29).

Figure 3.25: Frame

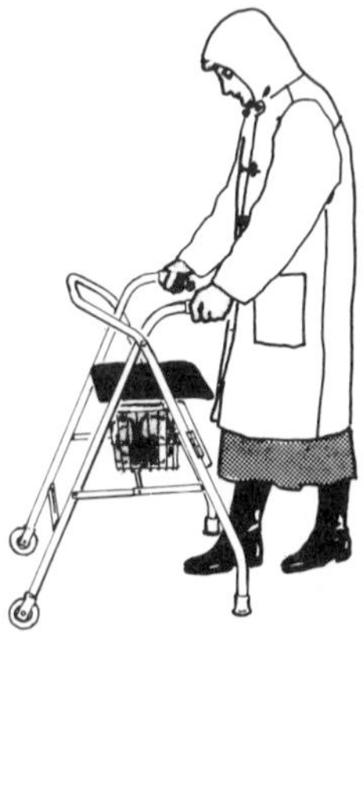

Figure 3.26: Metco Walkabout — Walking Frame with Basket and Brakes

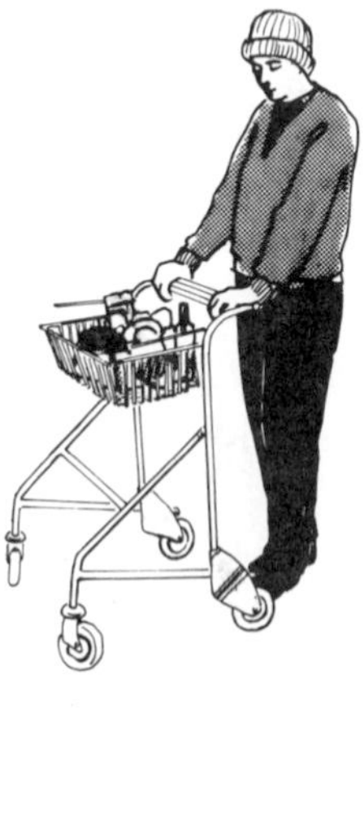

Figure 3.27: Single-handed Tray

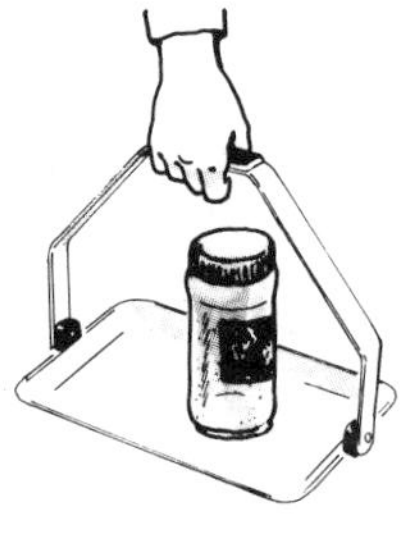

Figure 3.28: Swing Tray

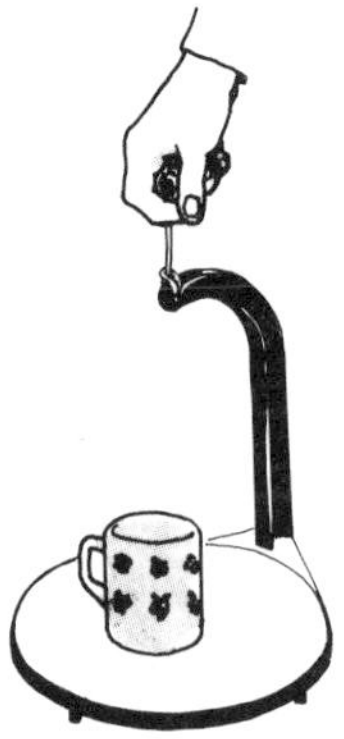

Figure 3.29: Dycem Freehand Tray

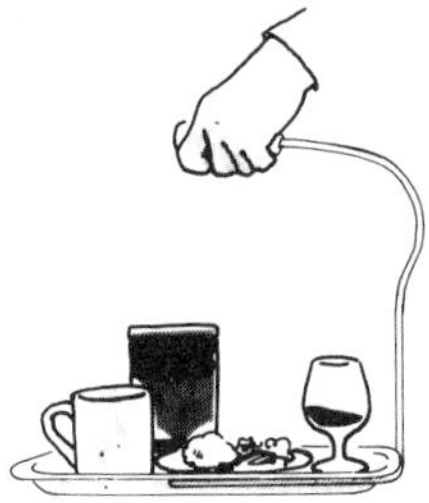

Lap Trays

Wheelchair users (and anyone who prefers to work with a tray on their lap) might like to consider the lap tray, which has no rim but is padded underneath with a cushion filled with polystyrene beads. This cushion automatically shapes itself over the thighs making it steady at whatever angle it is placed on the lap. Since the surface is fairly slippery it might be wise to add slip-resistant material before use (see Holding and Steadying, p. 64-5). A ledge at one side of the surface enables the tray to be used as a desk and also stops things sliding off to that side. The padding also makes it easier to carry hot items.

Other Trays

Most wheelchair manufacturers make trays to fit their models but these trays are not interchangeable. However, trays are available to fit onto most designs of wheelchair and some only onto one side of the chair so that the tray can be swung aside or folded down.

Other Ideas for Carrying/Lifting

1. A vegetable rack on wheels or castors will carry many things besides vegetables. The racks can be bought ready-made, some with removable baskets, some not.
2. Milk bottle carriers are also useful for other bottles or glasses. The safest type is the one with a fairly close grid at the bottom. One has a long-handled carrier to save bending down.
3. A plastic bucket (square or round) is safer and easier to carry than a bowl and liquids are less likely to spill out.
4. Many people find it useful to keep one basket at the bottom of the stairs and another at the top so that small items can be carried all at once whenever anyone is going up or down. It is possible to buy a household tidy, or a tool box, which is a divided plastic box on a handle like a basket.
5. If all the items necessary to do a job (say shoe cleaning) are kept in a plastic holder with pockets, the job becomes much easier. The bag or holder can be hung on the back of a cupboard door and taken to wherever the job is to be done.
6. A hinged ramp fitted to the side of a trolley can be placed with its other end on an oven shelf or worktop so that dishes can be slid to and fro rather than lifted (see p. 83).
7. Aprons with large pockets are useful. Apron (waist) 'hoops' eliminate the need to tie the strings. Cloth Kits sell a good sized apron with pockets already cut out and ready to sew. It is as well to bear in mind that plastic aprons are inclined to melt if placed too near heat.

Serving a Meal

Especially when entertaining, consider how to keep the food warm, and how it will be carried to table and served on to plates. Short-cuts help, for instance, potatoes baked in their jackets, cooking in oven-to-table ware and using a microwave cooker.

It is also easier to set out at least one of the courses, for example, salads arranged on the plate or bowl, sweets made in individual dishes, all in your own time.

People are quite willing to serve themselves — with the possible exception of carving a joint (and even that can be delegated).

Tongs, palette knives, straining spoons and soup ladles might be of more use than ordinary tablespoons. Flan knives with retractable pushers can help to slide a slice of cake or tart on to a plate.

The various kinds of tongs available have different attributes. Spring-handled tongs might be stiff for those with weak grip, but the spaghetti type, with teeth on them, have a firm grip particularly useful to blind people although they might damage soft items (Figure 3.30). Spring tongs with flat spatula ends are no use for handling rounded items (for instance, potatoes, root vegetables).

Figure 3.30: Spaghetti Tongs

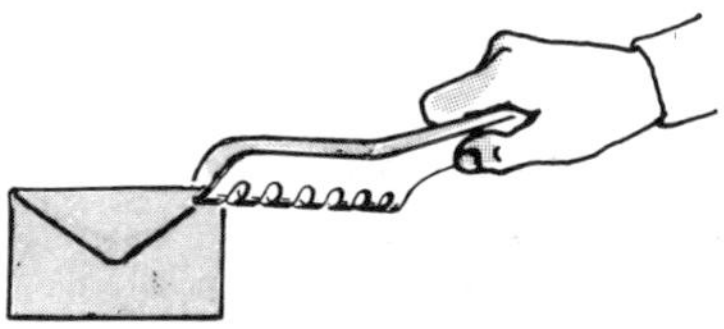

Light tongs with scissor handles lift small items efficiently, but might be difficult to manipulate. 'Duetto' tongs, with no spring, can be opened wider than those which have a spring. They can be separated into two spatulas and can be assembled with the curved spatula ends facing the same way. 'Stirex' kitchen tongs have a heatproof plastic loop handle with a gentle spring action; scissor handles are also incorporated.

Keeping Food Warm

By using a trolley and/or hatch, the cook can cut down the time taken to get the food to the table (see 'Carrying Things', p. 90). Thermos containers can be used to hold stews and soup. An electric warming tray is a good investment, or a table heater (some heated by night lights). Also, heated trolleys are available, which are designed on the same principle as the warming tray (see Chapter 2, p. 45).

Carving

The sharper the knife, the easier the job. There are cheap and efficient sharpeners on the market. A carving tray with spikes helps to hold the meat steady, while a knife with a handle set at right angles to the blade (Figure 3.16) used in conjunction with a similarly designed fork (Figure 3.31) to hold the meat, will help those with weak grip.

Electric carving knives make carving easier, but before buying one make sure that you can hold and operate it easily (see Chapter 2).

Eating

Holding and handling cutlery can be a difficult task especially for anyone with poor grip, with weak or stiff arms or who has only one hand. (See also Chapter 5, 'Eating in Company'.)

Figure 3.31: Fork with Right-angled Grip

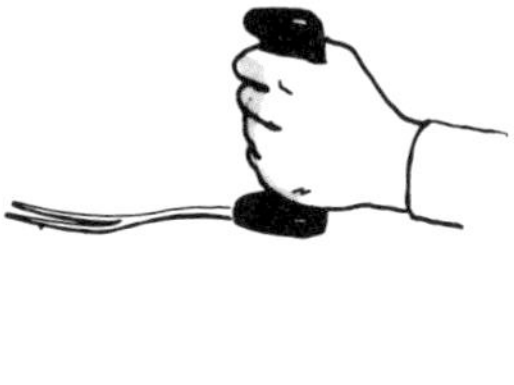

Weak Grip

Several ranges of cutlery have handles that are easier to hold because they are larger than standard size. It is worth looking at these ranges, as the handles may be large enough to be gripped without further 'padding'.

If a broader grip is required, several specially designed ranges of cutlery are available, some with interchangeable handle grips and one with an extra handstrap for even greater stability (Figure 3.32(a),(b), and (c)). Various kinds of 'padding' — sponge rubber tubing which can be cut to the required length (Figure 3.33) or a moulding plastic which can be shaped to the exact grip of the user — can be attached to handles (Figure 3.34). The latter sticks to one handle and is not therefore interchangeable with other cutlery.

Some people who find it difficult to cut food buy the ingredients already cut up, for instance, packs of stewing meat and mince in the supermarket, or mince it themselves; boneless joints can be cut with a 'Dux' knife. It is also possible to buy cartons of pre-cut salads and pre-grated cheese. Some foods (such as fish) are easier to eat with a fork.

One-handed Cutlery

There are several 'combined' pieces of cutlery; the range should be considered carefully before one type is chosen. One of these is the Nelson knife (Figure 3.35) which is designed like a cheese knife; it has a curved rocker blade with prongs at the end of the blade for spiking pieces of food. Although there is a danger that the wide sharp blade will be put into the

Figure 3.32a: Dorsal Wrist Splint to Hold Utensils

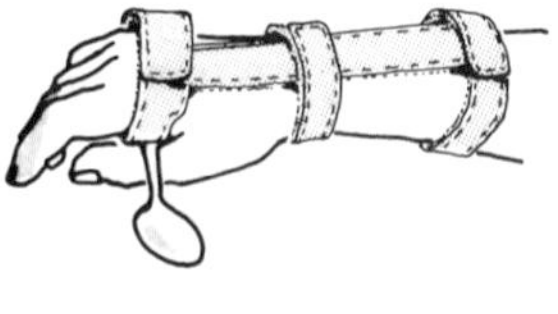

Figure 3.32b: Plastic Utensil Handclip

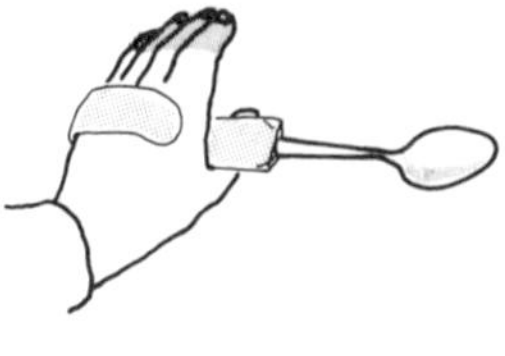

Figure 3.32c: Handstrap for Utensils

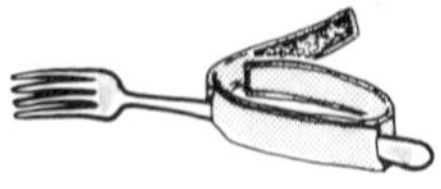

Figure 3.33: Plastazote Tubing to Enlarge Grip

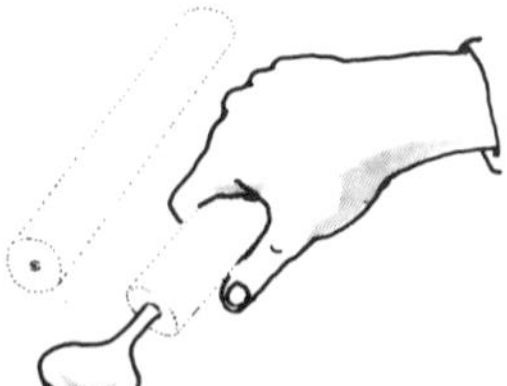

Figure 3.34: U2 Form Individually Moulded Grips

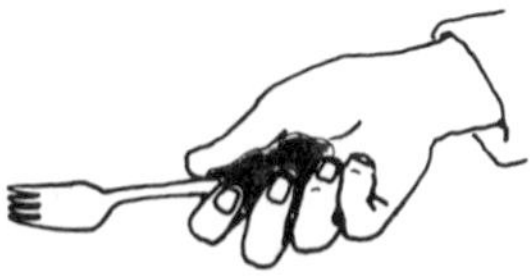

Figure 3.35: Nelson Knife Combined Knife and Fork

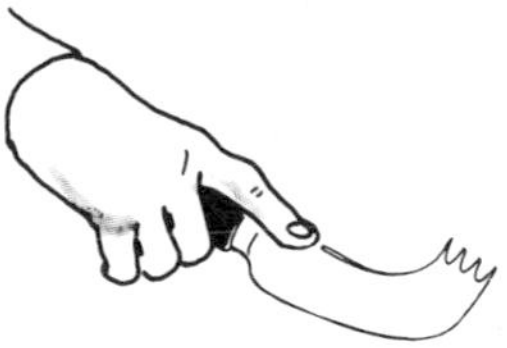

mouth while the fork is being used, some people find this knife useful because the cutting edge is sharp. Others prefer a standard cheese knife because the blade is narrower. The advantage of both these blades is the rocking facility — possibly the easiest way to cut for one-handed people. There is a rocking knife (Figure 3.36) with an easy-grip handle which cuts particularly efficiently.

The Manoy knife, less obviously 'different' than the Nelson, has a rocker blade useful for one-handed people to cut up food.

Some of the other types of 'combined' cutlery have cutting edges that are not sharp enough to cut meat but are therefore safer to use and look, like a Manoy, more like ordinary cutlery (Figure 3.37).

Plates

A guard to fit onto a plate gives the person eating something to push against, while a special oval shaped plate with a sloping base and an indent built into the rim prevents food sliding off the plate. When food is pushed against the undercut, it turns the food on to the spoon or fork. The plastic

Figure 3.36: Amefa Knife

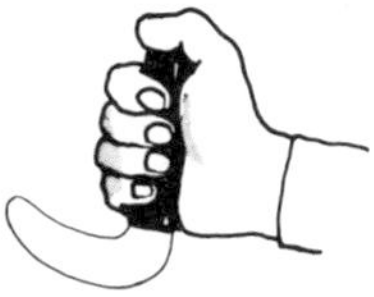

Figure 3.37: Knork (Combined Knife and Fork) and Knoon (Combined Fork and Spoon)

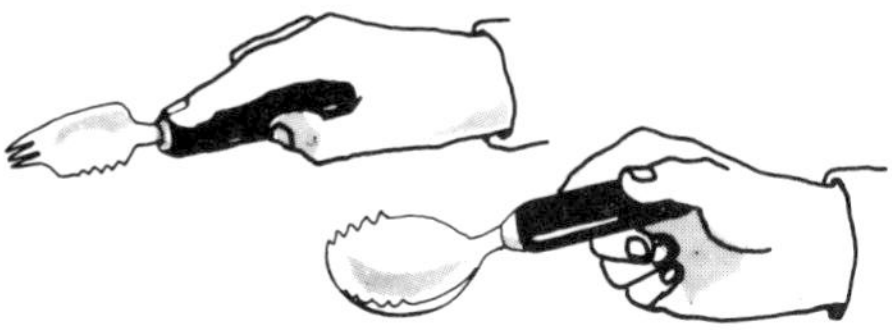

Manoy plates incorporate this feature as does the Royal Doulton 'Steelite 80' range (earthenware). While the latter plates are less obtrusive than a guard, a guard can more easily be taken on holiday or when eating away from home although some hotels provide the Steelite range (and it is always worth asking). Another alternative is to use a soup plate instead of an ordinary dinner plate.

Anyone who is visually handicapped (that is, using residual vision) should try to purchase both dark and light coloured plates so that whatever food is being eaten, its colour contrasts with that of the plate. A contrasting dark or light line (depending on the colour of the crockery) round the edge of a plate can also be useful.

Stiff Wrists

Angled cutlery may be helpful — the principle being that the spoon or fork is already turned towards the mouth when it is lifted from the plate. Anyone considering buying this type of cutlery should try it out first to make sure that it is set at the right angle. Counterbalanced spoons might also be considered (see below).

Tremor

It is possible to obtain counterbalanced spoons which stay level no matter at what angle the handle is held. Try these out first because tremor problems vary so much.

Lifting Food to the Mouth

If this is a problem:

1. use a high table (or a low chair) and rest your arm on the table;
2. use an arm support (which might have to be specially made, see p. 83); either fixed to the table on a screw clamp or as a sling hung from above on a frame or from the ceiling. Alternatively, simply use an upturned biscuit tin for support or put the plate on a tin to raise it;
3. ball-bearing arm supports are multi-adjustable 'gutter' supports attached to a wheelchair, and are obtainable to fix to a chair through the DHSS (if the chair was issued by the DHSS);
4. some people rest one arm on the table and bend the head to the plate so that the arm need not be lifted;
5. long-handled cutlery can be constructed with an interlocking system, so that the cutlery handle is fitted together at any angle or length to suit the user.

If Metal Cutlery Hurts the Mouth

Some ranges of picnic cutlery are made of hard-wearing, lightweight plastic with smooth edges.

Drinking

Many of those who dislike the mugs made specially for disabled people prefer a cup or mug with a large handle, although these can be heavy to lift. From the wide range of pottery mugs available it should be possible to find one that is suitable. An alternative is an insulated cup which is light and also keeps the drink hot.

People with weak or shaky hands often find it easier to drink from cups with two handles. These are usually plastic, sometimes with a spouted lid. Large (but heavy) two-handled pottery mugs are made by Royal Doulton in their 'Steelite 80' range in various patterns. Also, two-handled soup cups, if obtainable in the same pattern as the rest of the teaset, will look less conspicuous than a special two-handled mug. Cups or mugs with a contrasting line around the rim and along the handle may be easier for visually handicapped people.

'Do-it-yourself' handles can be: (1) interchangeable handles on 'girdles' that fit round the cup or mug; (2) handle-making kits, similar to modelling clay, that can be stuck to the sides of the drinking vessel in any shape or width (Figure 3.38). This can be used to make a second handle on a standard item.

Mugs with spouts are normally designed for children, but adult sizes are now available. Usually made of plastic, they can be disposable on a two-handled holder with a spouted lid, or a beaker with or without handles (Figure 3.39).

Special cups include the Manoy beaker with a shape in the base to fit the hand (Figure 3.40). These beakers are therefore difficult to drop and the shaped base is easier to hold than a handle — they can be supported by someone with almost no grip at all.

Figure 3.38: Grip-kit Moulded Grip

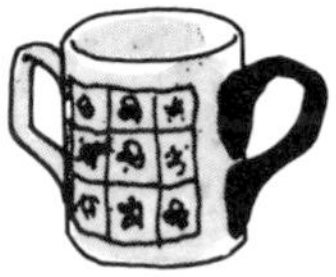

Figure 3.39: Selectagrip System with Choice of Cup and Handles

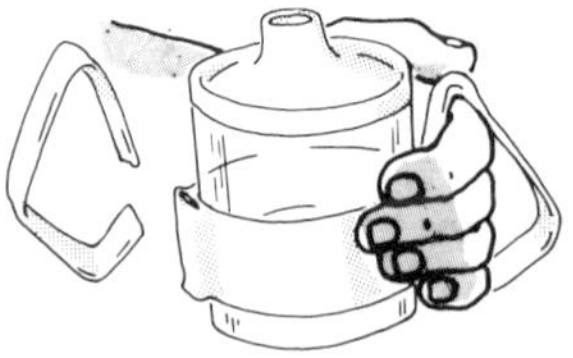

Figure 3.40: Manoy Beaker

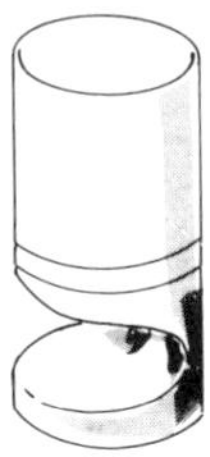

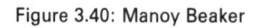

Straws of the following types are available:

1. Flexistraws which are tougher than ordinary straws and have a pleated section so that they can be angled (Figure 3.41).
2. Plastic tubing which can be obtained from wine-making departments in general stores or chemists.
3. Glass tubing which can be ordered in the surgical department of Boots the chemist. Although glass is fragile, many people prefer it because, unlike plastic, it has no taste.
4. A special plastic straw with a non-return valve prevents liquid returning down the straw. This is particularly helpful for people who cannot maintain sucking power.

Glasses and tumblers are often easier to handle if they have a heavy base, and are more likely to be seen by visually handicapped people if they are made of tinted glass.

Unbreakable plastic tumblers (made of polycarbonate) are sometimes preferred by anyone likely either to drop things or to bite the rim by accident.

Figure 3.41: Flexistraw with Clip Holder

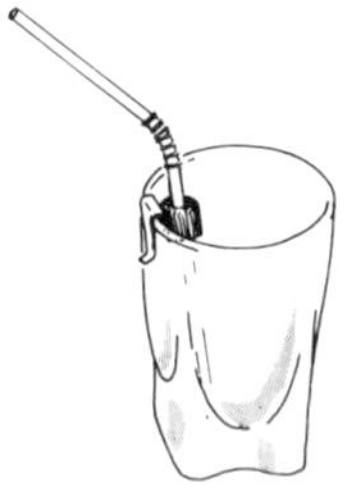

Boiling Water

See Chapter 2, p. 43 for electric free-standing and wall-hung kettles. Before buying a non-electric kettle, check that it stands firmly and that you can fill it easily (some kettles are filled through the spout). Always buy a good quality kettle for safety reasons.

Some people use a mini immersion heater which heats just the mug of water it is placed in, while others boil a cup or two of water in a small egg saucepan.

Making and Serving Tea. Teabags make the teapot easier to clean and are easier to dispose of than tealeaves. They can also be put straight into the cup for a single cup of tea and removed with either a teaspoon or special 'teabag tongs'.

A tea dispenser fixed on the wall cuts out the need for opening canisters or packets and measuring with the spoon. A one-cup infuser saves the bother of using a teapot. A thermal plastic teapot keeps the tea hot and is light to lift. A visually handicapped person could fill the pot (from the tap) with water and then pour this into the kettle; the amount of water boiled is therefore exact, so cutting down the risk of scalding when the teapot is filled with boiling water. The new tall, narrow electric kettles need only a cupful of water to cover the element.

If you have difficulty in lifting a teapot or kettle, there are two kinds of teapot stand designed to tip the pot without lifting. They are safe to use and there is no need to hold the handle when tipping the pot, although it is probably safer to put a hand on the lid (Figure 3.42a).

Tippers are also designed for standard kettles (not the jug type) which have an added balance or spring so that the kettle returns to the level position if released at any stage (Figure 3.42b). Even when being filled the kettle need not be lifted, since it can be filled either with a jug or by using a hose on the tap. Remember that the heaviest part of the kettle is the water inside it — boil only as much water as you need at the moment. Some find the type of teapot that has a handle over the top, like a kettle, easier both to lift and tilt, while wall-hung water heaters save lifting the kettle. Jug-type kettles are comparatively lightweight and have large handles which make them easier to tip (see Chapter 2, p. 44).

Making Coffee

One of the easiest ways to make ground coffee is to put the coffee in a warmed jug and pour boiling water on, as for tea. Coffee bags and individual coffee filters are easy to use and save mess, and a single cup can be made with one bag or filter; however, opinions vary as to the quality of the coffee produced. Filter coffee is almost as easy to make as the simple method outlined above, and can be obtained in ready-packed individual filters. Instant powdered or granulated coffee is popular and convenient.

Choose a coffee pot carefully: consider the size of handle, weight of pot

Figure 3.42a: Wooden Teapot Tipper

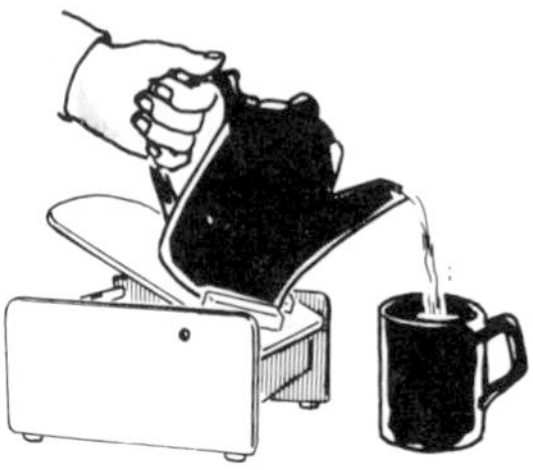

Figure 3.42b: Sunflower Kettle Tipper

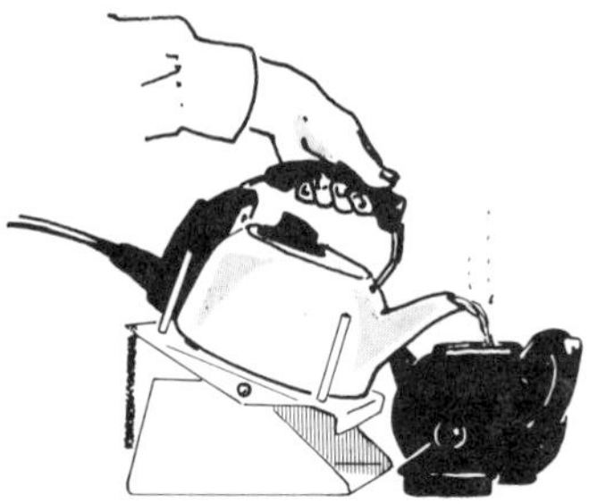

and type of lid. Enamel or stainless steel coffee pots are lighter than pottery ones and often have a hinged lid, but not all have easy-to-grasp handles. Alternatively, a stainless steel teapot could be used for making coffee, although some people think metal pots give coffee a bitter taste.

Coffee Makers. If considering an electric coffee maker, remember to review the *whole* operation (assembling, lifting, using, dispensing, cleaning) before buying. Not all these machines make coffee hot enough to suit all tastes (see Chapter 2, p. 44).

Waste Disposal

Disposing of waste in the kitchen can be made easier if a supply of used plastic or paper bags is kept near each work centre (for instance, the sink) into which waste can be thrown immediately, and later transferred to the bin. A waste bin lined with a polythene or strong paper bag will prevent the bin itself from being soiled. If the bag is tied when full, it will not smell if it has to wait to be disposed of.

The most common types of waste bin are those with a foot pedal or swing-top. The big swing-top bins are easy to open and a useful height (no need to bend), but when full the liner may be heavy and awkward to lift out.

Another alternative is to put the rubbish into a bag fixed to a frame at a chosen height on the kitchen wall or onto a cupboard door. Similar units have a heat-sealing device which closes the bag completely ready for putting into the bin.

Some sinks incorporate a waste disposal unit which macerates most *soft* material (but not tins or bottles) before they are washed away. These are noisy, but very convenient for vegetable peelings, fat and so on (see p. 20).

Cleaning up the Kitchen

In appropriate sections in this book, reference is made to cleaning procedures for different appliances and surfaces. However, there are one or two general guidelines which may be worth considering by someone who has recently become disabled or at any time when cleaning becomes just too much.

1. Do not let it get you down! Do not feel 'I *must* do it'. Why must you? The dirt will soon accumulate again and it won't do anybody any harm. Just tackle the jobs which worry *you* most — never mind about 'what other people may think'. Cleaning is a most dull and repetitive chore, not creative like cooking, and when it also becomes painful, it's time to leave it!
2. If you are very houseproud, work out a simple routine to follow (a) daily and (b) weekly. This book is concerned only with the kitchen, but

similar rules apply elsewhere in the house. A simple representative plan might run as follows:

daily — wipe over the cooking hob and all cooking surfaces after cooking. If you cannot see very well, plan a sequence to follow each day so that you do not miss anywhere and remember back edges and corners. Wash up only once a day;

weekly — wipe taps, door knobs, cupboard doors and so on. Clean splashes off toaster, kettle, sink and other chrome articles. Clean kitchen floor;

monthly — clean paint work, windows and shelves, but only if they need it.

3. Keep up-to-date with new cleaning materials and 'gadgets'. A really acceptable present would be an escorted trip, plus gift tokens, to a big hardware department or store to see what is on offer and stock up on items which would help most. It is difficult to recommend specific items as they not only vary over the country (as small local factories bring out new lines) but may equally well be withdrawn from sale, quite understandably, if they do not achieve commercial success. Mail order firms usually offer a wide range of ideas.

4. It is not necessary to have a lot of different cleaning agents — general purpose ones save getting mixed up. A good liquid cream cleanser which cleans most surfaces and a suitable floor cleaning liquid may be all you need — plus, of course, a washing-up liquid and favourite laundry products.

Beware of aerosols if your sight is not so good as it is easy for anyone to mix them up. Make sure the ones you like to use are really clearly labelled.

Useful Tips

The following help towards easier cleaning.

1. Easy-to-clean work tops.
2. Open shelves of wood painted or covered with adhesive plastic.
3. Cupboard shelves or drawers lined with paper or adhesive plastic sheeting.
4. Cupboard doors painted with extra hard gloss paint to stand up to constant wiping.
5. Flooring which does not show marks and only requires easy cleaning.
6. Cooker and refrigerator on lockable castors or special castor base for occasional moving; if they are flat on the floor, accept that there is no need to move them out at all.
7. The floor clear of baskets, stools, bins and so on; store off the floor if possible (a vegetable rack on castors is useful).
8. Work tops clear of unnecessary articles.
9. A baking tray or roasting tin under casseroles or pie dishes in the oven to catch drips.

10. Meat cooked in covered dish, foil, or cooking bag to avoid fat spots in the oven.
11. All spills on cooker (milk, vegetable water, and so on) wiped up as they happen — keep a clean cloth handy for this purpose.
12. Fat stains removed when cooker is warm.
13. Kitchen kept well ventilated.
14. Spills on the floor wiped up as they happen.
15. All materials for a particular job, for instance, cooker cleaning, kept in a plastic box or basket near at hand.
16. Have only equipment you really use.

Tackling the Various Jobs

Many commercial products make the job of keeping the kitchen clean easier. If their initial expense deters you, consider their value to you, how long they will last and whether one piece of equipment could not be used for several jobs, for example, a sponge mop will clean floors, walls and windows.

Floor Cleaning

Try to sit down to do this job. First, remove loose dirt with a long-handled brush and dustpan, or vacuum cleaner, and then, using a hose, fill a bucket (rectangular shape is useful) quarter-full while it is on the floor. Using a sponge mop and proprietary cleaner, clean the floor. A piece of nylon scourer under the sponge will remove stubborn stains. If you wish to have a shine on the floor, finish with a special slip-resistant preparation by putting a cloth under the squeezed out sponge mop. (See Chapter 3, p. 88 for specific tips for those who find it difficult to bend.)

If you have a carpet in the kitchen, studies suggest that a cylinder, rather than an upright, vacuum cleaner is easier for most disabled people. Very lightweight upright cleaners are, however, available if these seem easier to handle; for instance, the small cleaners designed for cleaning stairs can be bought with an extension tube.

There are so many types of cleaners (for instance, easy to pull along; audible signal when dust-bag is full) that the only solution is to go to a shop and examine them before choosing the one that suits you best.

Cleaning the Cooker

See Chapter 2, p. 31.

Care of Refrigerator and Freezer

See pp. 48-52.

Care of the Sink

Fill the sink with hot water and proprietary cleaner and leave to soak — finish the job with a dish mop. Draining boards need wiping regularly, and, if they are stainless steel, drying to prevent water marks. A cream cleanser removes stains.

Working Surface Cleaning

Uncluttered surfaces are easier to keep clean. Use a dish mop to reach the back. Dry with mutton cloth or other dry cloth.

Window Cleaning

Use a spray cleaner for windows. This is easy to apply from a distance (a clear one leaves no marks if you miss a bit!). Clean off with a sponge mop with an angled sponge.

4 Healthy Eating

Creina Murland

Food is enjoyable and eating is a pleasurable occupation. Food 'does you good' but, because that phrase has been a commonplace to most people from childhood, all too many adults have tended to overlook this fact and to eat only foods they like or which are easy to prepare, sometimes with unfortunate repercussions on their health.

In the last decade or two, nutritional research has been going on and the more startling disclosures have been headlined, leading to a reverse swing in the attention given to food. Thinking people have become concerned, even frightened, about their food intake, which has led to slimming crazes and to fad diets.

Now, at last, there is plenty of sane thinking and advice available. All the scientific thinking and terminology is there, well documented for the professional to study (see Appendix III) but for the layman, the concern has been replaced with sensible, practical guidelines which bring back the fun to eating. By following a few easy-to-remember guidelines, you can rest assured that you are eating healthy food, in correct proportions, for day-to-day fitness. Some disabled people will need to adapt these guidelines but, in general, the new thinking suits everybody. Fortunately, this gentle revolution coincides with an increasing interest in natural foods, now available in a wide range of shops.

First, let us have a reminder about the main groups of food, and a description of the different jobs they do in the body, followed by an indication of the relative proportions in which you are advised to eat them.

The golden rule for healthy eating is variety. A simple scheme is to divide foods into groups and to eat a small selection of foods from each group every day:

1. milk and milk products (Figures 4.1 and 4.2);
2. meat and alternatives — cheese, eggs, fish, poultry, peas, beans and lentils;
3. fruit and vegetables (Figures 4.3 and 4.4);
4. bread and cereals (Figures 4.5 and 4.6).

Each of these groups contain certain nutrients which are essential to maintain life, to protect the body from illness and to aid recovery from illness and bodily disorders. These nutrients are sometimes found in more than one group, which can be confusing. Do not worry about them, simply refer to the list below from time to time to check advice and remember that

Figures 4.1 and 4.2: Milk, Milk Products and Protein Foods

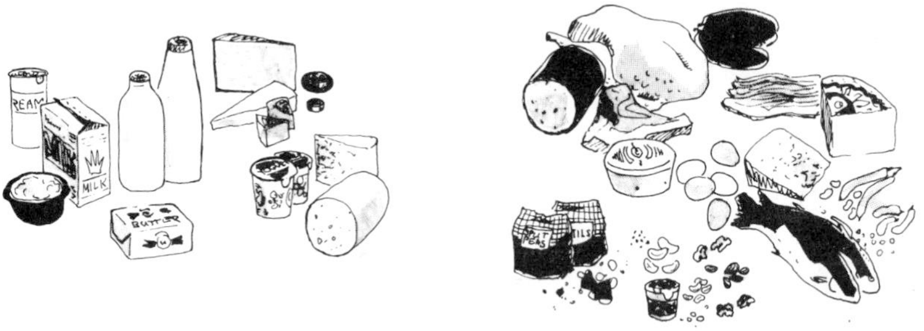

Figures 4.3 and 4.4: Vegetables and Fruit

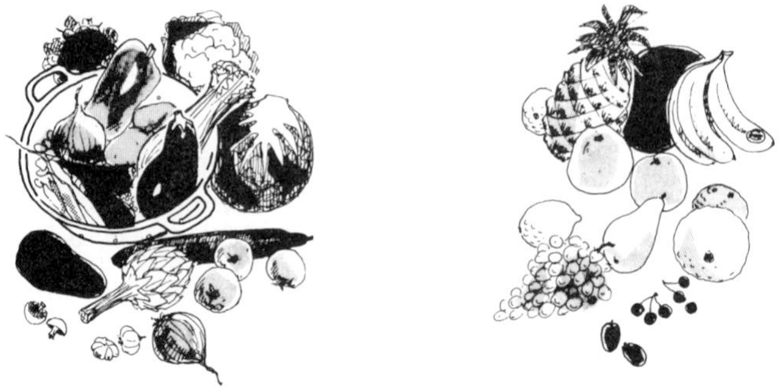

Figures 4.5 and 4.6: Bread, Cereals and Liquids

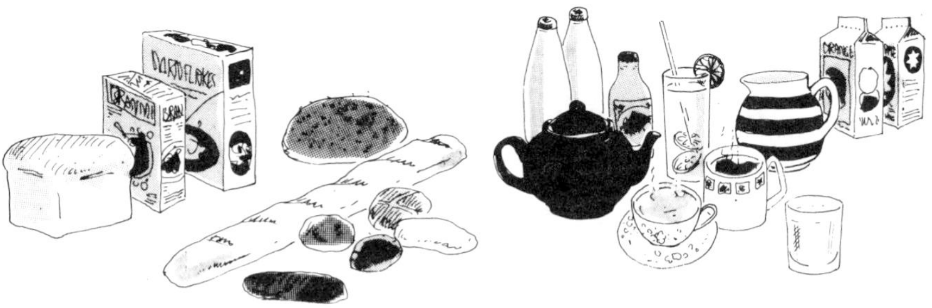

a moderate quantity from each of the main food groups will ensure that your body is getting what it needs, while you just enjoy eating it.

Main Nutrients

The main nutrients contained in food are: protein, fat, carbohydrate, vitamins, mineral salts and water.

Protein

Protein is used for growth, for the repair of tissues and for the maintenance of body processes, and all this can only occur if the need for energy is fully met. Some examples of protein are: (1) animal sources — milk, meat, fish, eggs, cheese; (2) vegetable sources — flour and flour products, cereals, nuts, pulse vegetables — peas, beans, lentils. A mixture of animal and vegetable protein is of greatest value.

Fat

Fat is used as a concentrated source of energy. Some fats also carry fat-soluble vitamins. Fat is either animal or vegetable in origin. Some examples are: (1) animal fats — butter, cream, whole milk, cheese, egg yolk, lard, oily fish; (2) vegetable fats — nuts, most margarines, cooking oils.

Carbohydrate

All carbohydrate, except cellulose, gives energy. Sugars, starch and cellulose all belong to this group. Some examples are: (1) containing sugar — all types of sugar and foods made with it, for instance, biscuits, sweetened fizzy drinks; jam, marmalade, syrup, honey; all fruit (varying amounts); (2) containing starch — all cereals, potatoes, pulse vegetables; (3) containing cellulose or fibre — fruit, vegetable, wholegrain cereals.

Fibre. Fibre is necessary to assist bowel action because it passes through the body unchanged. An increased intake of fibre and fluid to prevent constipation is preferable to habitual use of laxatives. Some examples of good sources of fibre are: wholemeal bread, bran type breakfast cereals, baked jacket potatoes, baked beans, bananas.

Vitamins

These substances, which are present in small amounts in food, are essential for various functions in the body. Named after letters of the alphabet, two of these all important substances are of particular importance to disabled and elderly people.

Vitamin C. This is important to prevent bruising, bleeding gums and as an essential aid to the healing of broken skin. It is a water-soluble vitamin which is very easily destroyed by prolonged storage, soaking and over-cooking of vegetables and fruit. The main sources are citrus fruits, summer berry fruits, green vegetables, potatoes (especially new), tomatoes.

Vitamin D. Vitamin D works in conjunction with calcium and phosphorus. It is especially important for elderly people to have an adequate intake to prevent their bones becoming brittle. In addition to food sources of this vitamin, a major source is sunshine and ultraviolet light. Main sources are margarine, butter, eggs, oily fish.

Mineral Salts

These are also present in small amounts in food and either help to form body tissues or fluids or help in chemical reactions. Examples of mineral salts include calcium, iron and sodium.

Calcium. This is for formation of bones and teeth. An adequate intake of calcium is especially important for older people who may develop brittle bones. Good sources of calcium are milk, cheese and green vegetables.

Iron. This forms part of the red blood cells which carry oxygen. Anaemia (lack of iron) may cause lethargy and tiredness. Good sources of iron are meat, green vegetables and eggs.

Sodium. This is an essential part of all body fluids and common salt is the largest single source. Even so, some of us tend to take too much salt, so moderation is the keyword here, too. As it is present in numerous prepared and processed foods, try not to add too much to food on the plate.

By trying to eat something from each of the main food groups each day, you are automatically getting some of each of the main nutrients as well. However, remember that too much of some foods are too much of a good thing, so try to balance them with each other for a healthy diet. A high proportion of meat and dairy foods, for instance, could lead to an excess of fat. Not eating any vegetables or fruit could lead to a serious shortage of vitamin C. As a nation, the British tend to indulge these two failings. Similarly, fats and carbohydrates are essential for warmth and energy but people who cannot be active enough to use up that energy intake, for one reason or another, will tend to keep it as excess weight.

No Drastic Change Needed

Change does not always need to be drastic. Generally speaking, most people need to eat daily:

1. some meat or alternatives — cheese, eggs, fish, poultry, peas, beans, lentils;
2. some milk and milk products;
3. less fats and oils;
4. less sugar and salt;
5. more bread, cereals and potatoes;
6. more vegetables and fruit.

Such a change of emphasis could also have some happy side-effects. It is likely that the amount of money spent on food would be less; the incidence of high blood pressure and related disorders would decrease, and the inclusion of more cellulose (which used to be known as roughage and is now called fibre) appears to be beneficial.

Liquids

Water. Water is essential for all body processes, and the importance of an adequate intake of water or other fluids of which water forms a part is not always realised. About 1.7 litres (3 pints) daily is the recommended amount, but this can be made up easily by the normal intake of tea, coffee, milky drinks, soups and cold unsweetened fruit drinks, which we enjoy at different times of the year, and by remembering that all foods contain a certain amount of water.

Alcohol. Small amounts of alcohol (unless there are medical contra-indications) can be beneficial to stimulate appetite, increase circulation and aid sleep. The social value of alcohol is important and a drink and a friendly chat is a useful way of entertaining. The stronger spirits are not always necessary and many people enjoy the gentler delights of the fashionable aperitifs, cocktails and low-calorie mixer drinks. However, alcohol is expensive and can be addictive — and it is not essential.

Planning Ahead

Some of the many publications based on this new easier way of planning healthy eating are listed in Appendix III. They will help you to rethink your eating habits, if necessary, and a little forethought will make things easier. Without being too rigid, it is possible to plan ahead, probably weekly, what you will eat each day, at least for the main meal of the day. This is not only nutritionally sound, it is also practical, as it helps with budgeting and shopping (see Chapters 6 and 7).

Most people keep a small stock of dry goods in a cupboard, augmented with canned foods and possibly some frozen ones. So only fresh foods, such as meat, vegetables and bread, need to be bought weekly. Top up stores as required, weekly or monthly, and then buy a selection of meat or fish as needed, plus fruit and vegetables. Vary what you buy according to season.

Although at least one cooked meal a day is comforting and cheering, do not worry if you don't feel like cooking. A cold meal is just as nutritious. Very often a quickly made hot drink or soup will perk up a cold meal. Similarly, do not despise the humble sandwich — easy, quick and sustaining. Well-chosen, commercially prepared foods can also be invaluable and can be just as nutritious. Read the labels first, if you can, to ascertain the ingredients.

Individual Adjustments

Although most people can follow the foregoing recommendations quite easily, others are advised by their doctors to lose weight, to gain it or even to avoid certain groups of foods altogether. In these cases, a little more thought and planning is necessary, plus an acceptance that previous bad eating habits may have contributed to the present situation.

Overweight

As many disabled people cannot be as active as they would wish and may even, albeit subconsciously, eat more to cheer themselves up, overweight is probably one of the most common nutritional problems with which they have to contend, and obesity may lead to undue strain on the heart, lungs, joints and muscles. Excess weight may also be due to fluid retention and, if this occurs, seek advice from your doctor.

The information in the previous pages applies to overweight people, of course, but from the outset it is important to apply some new thinking to the food plan, and stick to it.

1. Accept that lack of exercise can contribute to weight problems and, if you cannot do even gentle exercise, then cut down what you eat overall, but especially oils and fats.
2. Little meals and often, eaten at regular times, are better than one or two big ones.
3. Don't cut out breakfast. A good, cereal-based breakfast is very important to give you a good start to the day.
4. Cut out all sugar and sugary foods and drinks, if possible. Sugar contains only carbohydrate and it tends to displace other more nutritious foods from the diet. Some of the newer, artificial sweeteners are excellent if you have a very sweet tooth.
5. Reduce the amount of fat eaten, both in the obvious ways and in less obvious ways. For instance, cut down on spreading fats — butter and margarines — and cut off all visible fat from meat. Consider using semi-skimmed milk (now very easily obtainable) instead of whole milk; eat less hard cheese and replace, if liked, with cottage cheese or other 'low fat' varieties; grill, bake, microwave, pressure cook or stew foods, according to kind, instead of frying them.
6. Choose leaner cuts of meat, or substitute fish, poultry or pulse vegetables for it. Remember that many meat products, such as sausages, pâté and corned beef, have a fairly high proportion of both fat and salt.
7. So-called 'slimming foods' are expensive and unnecessary. Also, if you eat a good varied diet, including plenty of fruit and vegetables, extra vitamin pills are not required.
8. If it breaks your heart to throw away dripping from roast or grilled meat, remember that birds love it and that you will be doing them a good

turn and giving yourself a lot of pleasure if you put it outside for them during the winter months.

Underweight

Here again, a moderate varied plan of healthy eating is better than concentrating only on fats and carbohydrates, although intake of these two groups can be stepped up. Protein-rich foods may help in rehabilitation after periods of illness — for instance, meat, fish and eggs.

In addition, if you don't feel much like eating during a period of convalescence, one of the fortified concentrated food products, taken in liquid form, can make a valuable addition to normal foods.

If you are either overweight or underweight, it is advisable to consult your doctor, health visitor or dietitian before embarking on a radical change in diet. But, for some special conditions, it is essential to plan your diet under medical and dietetic advice and supervision.

Skin Disorders

Modification of diet has an important role in the treatment and alleviation of certain skin conditions. Before embarking on any modifications, however, it is important that clinical tests are made to aid diagnosis and that individual special diets should be planned and followed only under medical and dietetic supervision. Certain forms of allergy and dermatitis are examples of conditions which can be helped by special diets. Irksome though they may be to follow, it is only wise to stick to them as recommended. Hospital clinics specialising in these conditions have dietitians who advise on treatment with, for example, gluten-free, low nickel and additive-free diets.

Other Medical Conditions

Modified diets are usually part of the recognised treatment for diabetes, heart conditions, kidney disorders, coeliac disease and other digestive or circulatory problems. In these cases, the diet is tailored to each individual's requirements and should be discussed in detail with the doctor and dietitian, who will endeavour to help on the practical side as well as with theoretical advice. Progress is monitored and the diet reviewed and adjusted from time to time as an ongoing part of the treatment. Certain dietary products are regarded as drugs and therefore available on prescription for specific conditions.

5 Eating in Company

Gwen Conacher

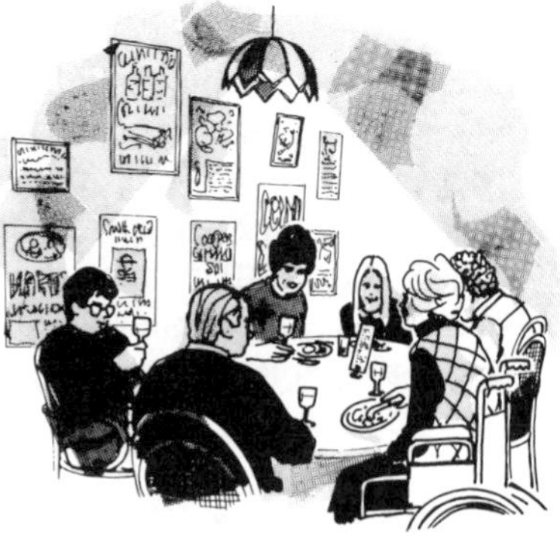

Eating is in itself a pleasure and many social contacts are made and maintained by eating together. Meetings of friends, family and colleagues are frequently planned around, and enhanced by, a meal, whether it is a snack or a banquet.

This very circumstance is sometimes an obstacle for disabled people to overcome — eating in company can be a real difficulty or imagined ordeal. But solitary eating, although a pleasant relaxation in itself, can get lonely if done all the time. One meal which is always pleasant on one's own is a leisurely breakfast. Plan to enjoy that, and don't miss this important meal.

Family partners and members or friends of long standing can give great support to anyone convalescing from a recent illness; they can also be a great help to each other as they grow older. People who find themselves alone after the family grows up and moves away, or through bereavement, may prefer their own company for a while, but eventually may wish to seek companionship and how better to do this than over a meal.

If you are naturally shy or are coping with a recent disablement, you may also prefer to eat at home for a while or to entertain a friend. In this case, there is no need to get worried about the actual provision of food. Several books have been written about cooking for one person or for two, on simple 'short-cut' cooking, or for those with limited mobility (see Appendix III). See also Chapter 7 for some easy ideas and recipes. You don't even have to cook at all — a simple sandwich or salad meal can be just as nourishing and attractive as hot meals, and can be prepared in advance so that you are not tired out when meeting a friend. And there is nothing wrong with having just a cup of tea or coffee, or a hot drink from a vacuum flask and a biscuit, as long as it is backed up later with a proper meal.

Community Services

Most local authorities, being well aware of the therapeutic value of eating in congenial company, offer a range of opportunities for eating with others. The actual arrangements vary from area to area; some facilities may be run by local social services departments, some by religious or social groups, others by voluntary, national or local organisations, but the types of service are similar. Ask your social worker or telephone the office of the Director of Social Services for your region, or the local Citizens' Advice Bureau (CAB), to find out which are available near your home.

Meals on Wheels

This service, although not strictly a version of 'community eating', is a helpful link between cooking all meals yourself and eating in company. 'MOW' is a service often run by social services with help from voluntary organisations, in particular the Womens' Royal Voluntary Service, which undertakes to deliver a hot, two-course meal to individual homes around lunch-time, for a small charge. It is principally for those over 60 and living alone, but can include disabled people in younger age groups. A doctor's recommendation is sometimes necessary. Preference is given to housebound or bedbound people or those otherwise unable to shop or cook for themselves. Similar temporary arrangements can usually be made during a period of illness or convalescence, if required. Special diets are available in some areas. Some London boroughs, for example, will provide kosher, Asian and vegetarian meals as well as medical diets.

The degree of help and the frequency of the service vary between areas. Meals are usually provided regularly, from one to five days a week, and some areas even make a weekend delivery.

Excellent as this service is, in your own interests you should try not to rely on it entirely, because if you supplement occasional meals on wheels deliveries with your own efforts you can help to maintain your health and well-being. Shopping gets you out of the house, keeps social contacts alive and gives you gentle exercise. Cooking, though it can be tiring, can be an enjoyable and creative activity which engages thoughts and concentration for part of each day.

Luncheon Clubs

Many luncheon clubs have been established in recent years, run by a number of different local organisations. Again, the social services, local disablement associations or CAB will have full details. Eligibility to join is sometimes related to the sponsoring body, but is usually only regulated by being of pensionable age. Some have transport available, usually free of charge, although a nominal charge is usually made for the two-course meal. Sometimes a short programme of games, music or a talk is arranged to follow the meal. Usually all the helpers are volunteers, and in some clubs the members are encouraged to take it in turns to help with running the club and serving the food.

Day Centres

Day centres may be run by social services as well as by voluntary organisations. All day can be spent at the centre, meeting friends for a chat, having coffee or tea as well as a main meal, and enjoying recreational facilities. People over pensionable age are eligible, as well as some disabled people of all ages, and transport is usually provided. In some cases, remedial care and occupational therapy are part of the service. The Office of the Director of Social Services can give details about local facilities.

Eating Out

Another step towards eating out in restaurants is to visit somewhere you know already: a small café or restaurant, a pub, or perhaps a pizza or hamburger bar.

First, however, you may like to break yourself in gently by sampling at home some of the interesting food available on a takeaway basis. This movement towards eating prepared food at home has grown rapidly and has a lot of advantages for disabled people.

Chinese, Indian and other national cuisines are available to take away at reasonable prices. Perhaps a friend can help with the logistics of buying the food and bringing it home. Some shops accept telephoned orders for collection and, in a few areas, shops will deliver the food. You will not have to cook it — sometimes you may not even have to heat it up. The food comes neatly packed in disposable containers, so there is no washing-up. Even the favourite British fish and chips or pie and chips are now classed as takeaways. New style 'chippies' also offer meals served on the premises, as do some of the other takeaway shops, so it may be a good idea to try food which is new to you in one of these unpretentious establishments so that you can get an idea of what to order to take home.

Younger readers, particularly, might feel more at ease in these informal restaurants and would also find the 'fast food' bars very accommodating. Go with friends who will help you. Although at first it may look frighteningly quick and efficient, you will find the slick style of service well thought out and easy to master. Although self-service is the rule, sometimes there is a member of staff to help you carry a tray and find you a seat.

Most public houses offer food with their drinks. Pubs make very good ports of call as almost all are easy of access, most have easily reached toilets (although perhaps not always adapted) and offer simple, good food at reasonable prices.

All these friendly eating places are also good stepping stones to what may be the final hurdle to many — lunching or dining in a luxury restaurant. Since the publication of the first edition of *Kitchen Sense*, considerable help and advice on this subject has been proffered by individuals and interested organisations, resulting in these guidelines on eating out for people with a wide range of disablement.

1. Without attempting to minimise the inherent difficulties, perhaps the first and most important point to bear in mind is that other people are probably not as conscious of your disability as you feel they are.
2. It is generally agreed that the troubles encountered when eating out are more than halved if you are with a friend. This should not be seen as a lack of independence, since for most of us much of the enjoyment of the meal is in the shared company. Many disabled people have experienced the comfort of being saved explanations by someone who will quietly find the right chair, order wine and the right shaped glass, or unobtrusively cut up the meat. This is especially true at a large celebration like a wedding or other party, particularly as this usually means facing an unfamiliar environment. A visually handicapped person will find a sighted friend invaluable in describing the lie of the land.
3. A little judicious homework helps tremendously. An advance telephone conversation with the manager of the restaurant you plan to visit can quickly establish the suitability of it from the point of view of access: Are there steps at the entrance, or on the way to the table? Is the door narrow, or at an angle? Are there swing or revolving doors to negotiate? Are the tables very close together? Are the seats 'fixed' or free-standing? Is there an adapted WC if you have a wheelchair?

Affirmative answers to any, or all, of these questions might mean that you have to think again about the venue, but if this is not possible, a request for assistance to reach the table will mean that someone will be prepared to help you on arrival. If you have a guide dog, check that it may come too. However, more and more restaurateurs are improving access to their premises, so presuming the answers to these first questions are favourable, you or your host should go on to explain that you will be arriving at a reasonably early hour (so you can get settled before most of the other customers come in) and that you would appreciate being placed at an easily reached table. If you use a wheelchair, ask if a chair can be removed at your place. Hotel restaurants are usually more spacious and accessible than specialist restaurants.
4. In most establishments, each of the above may be plain sailing, but the lavatories may be on another floor without a lift, difficult to locate or very small. These points should be checked if you are likely to need

toilet facilities during or after the meal.

5. If you lack co-ordination of movement or have to eat in a slightly unorthodox way, you may like to sit facing away from other tables.

6. If you normally use specialised eating aids or adapted cutlery, take them with you. Some disabled people do not like using them in company for fear of looking 'different'. But if you have learned to eat with special aids and eat better with them, it is worth considering whether or not it is more conspicuous to be eating comfortably with an aid than struggling with unfamiliar cutlery. It is also easy to slip a small piece of foam or a non-slip mat into your pocket or bag, if you usually use one.

7. If you cannot see very well, a number of helpful tips can be borne in mind — all submitted by visually handicapped people:

(a) when first seated at the table, quickly check the table setting by sitting close to the table edge and discreetly touching the handles of all the cutlery, and feeling where the glasses are. If you feel you might knock over a stemmed glass, don't hesitate to ask for a tumbler;

(b) have confidence to ask a companion, or the waiter, to read the menu to you slowly, so you can consider the alternatives and, for preference, choose something that does not need a lot of cutting up, such as steak, or which might slip on the plate, like melon, peas or lobster in its shell, or fish on the bone, for obvious reasons. Fish in sauce, dishes with rice, moussaka, goulash or similar foods which can be eaten with a fork and/or a spoon are easiest to tackle. Remember that most Far Eastern food is served in bite-sized pieces and meant to be eaten with a spoon. Salads can be tricky, unless the ingredients have been shredded and tossed together in a sauce;

(c) ask to have the condiment containers passed to you and described. Salt can be gently poured over a finger-tip to assess the quantity and rate of flow. Ask if the sugar is granulated or in lumps;

(d) ask your companion to describe the position of food on the plate, using the clock-face method;

(e) take the waiter into your confidence, ask him to speak to you before he is about to serve you, so you know where he is, and that the food is on its way to your plate. If you are the host, ask the waiter to tell you when he brings the bill, ask how much it is, and if service is included. Remember that the change may be returned to you on a plate, and again ask him to draw your attention to it.

Perhaps the last word in this section should be from a group of disabled students who regularly eat out in all the types of eating places discussed here. They assume that they will not meet any problems they cannot overcome and expect to be treated as ordinary customers — and they are!

6 Shopping

Gwen Conacher

Like it or loathe it, shopping for food is essential and must be undertaken by every homemaker, whether for a family or for just one or two people.

For disabled people who live with others, this may not be such a problem as it can be for the single person or even for two people, especially if both are elderly. When the first edition of this book was being compiled, enquiries revealed that 'shopping seems to present more difficulties for many disabled housewives than any other activity' and it was concluded that 'there are no easy answers to this problem'. Does that statement still hold good, some twelve years later?

Undoubtedly, in some parts of the country it still does. But it is equally true that there are many more facilities available now to ease the lot of the disabled shopper. Observance of the requirements of the Chronically Sick and Disabled Persons Act 1970 and the Disabled Persons Act 1981, though not mandatory, has ensured that new shops and supermarkets are being built with easier access, and public awareness of disablement has generally improved. Local government departments and voluntary organisations work continuously to improve the situation. Facility of transport to and from shopping areas has improved. Most of the big supermarket chains have done a lot to improve their stores ergonomically to everyone's advantage and offer a range of special amenities for disabled people. Unfortunately, as these stores are usually in big cities or large shopping centres, they favour those who live in large conurbations and, even for these people, sometimes involve a difficult journey.

Country dwellers may have to contend with less than convenient small shops and stores, but at least these are usually easier to reach and can offer more personal service.

A recent small survey conducted for this edition revealed more complaints about reaching the shops than actually using them. These problems do not really come within the remit of this book and conditions vary tremendously between areas. All disabled people are likely to have a helpful contact within the appropriate authority; something that everyone can do to help the community at large is to point out where there are shortcomings and ask for improvements to be made. Very often local authorities are not aware of what is needed but are only too happy to put things right once attention has been drawn to a local difficulty. People with visual handicaps are often the only ones who notice (often to their cost) the overhanging tree or projecting sign, an uneven pavement or a badly placed seat; they would be helping everyone if they would draw these hazards to the attention of those responsible or their social service contact.

It is difficult to give detailed advice and solutions to shopping problems as individual circumstances vary so much. However, there are a few general guidelines, based on helpful suggestions obtained from the survey, which are worth consideration. In addition, local access guides are usually obtainable. They are useful to newly disabled people or to new residents in a particular district. Ask about them from the social services department.

When to Shop

Most shops are busiest on Saturdays so try to shop during the week on a regular day which suits you. Weekly shopping trips make sense because they help you to plan and to budget carefully. They can well be linked with collecting a pension. However, if a weekly trip means a load which is too heavy to carry, then two or even three shopping trips a week may be easier. Some people who can walk reasonably well may even prefer to buy a few things each day, enjoying the exercise and social contact involved. At the other extreme, others arrange one big 'shop-in' each month, perhaps with the aid of a friend and just buy small quantities of perishable food as required.

Planning

However frequently you shop, it is always a good idea to take a shopping list to avoid forgetting something and to counteract temptation. Perhaps even more important than the shopping list, is the reminder list. Keep a pad and an attached pencil handy, so that as soon as something is used up it can be jotted down, ready to be replaced on the next shopping trip. This is particularly helpful for items used occasionally rather than regularly. A black felt-tipped marker pen on a marker board is suggested for those with impaired sight.

Try to keep a spare supply of essential items always in store so that in the event of bad weather or illness you are not badly inconvenienced if you run out. It is a good idea to replace the spare item as soon as it has been opened.

Some advisers recommend compiling a weekly menu and sticking to it, which may work for some but prove dull or irksome to others. This must be a personal choice. It can be a useful guide but, if adhered to strictly, allows no opportunity to take advantage of special offers.

Budgeting

Many frustrations and worries can be avoided by keeping to a carefully worked out household budget. It is generally recommended that expenditure on food and cleaning materials should amount to about one-third of the total income over a stated period — say, a month — always allowing sufficient for other essentials such as rent, rates, heating and clothes, plus a margin for incidentals like travel and presents. Individual circumstances mean that no two people will budget in the same way, but once you have decided on your plan try and stick to it.

Pennies can be saved (but it *is* only pennies) by comparing prices, using discount coupons for products you normally use and swapping those you don't want with other people. Special offers can be useful, but again, only on things you use regularly. As these are advertised in the windows of stores, it is not always easy for visually handicapped people to know what is available at any one time. Local broadcasting stations and local free press sometimes carry this information, as do talking newspapers. However, as the savings are small, don't be tempted into buying something you won't use before it becomes stale. Similarly, large size economy packs are not always economical for small families. On the other hand, supermarkets' own brand lines of basic foods are excellent value — good quality at reasonable prices.

In-store Information

Labelling of food packs has improved considerably. Unfortunately, because of the wealth of information required by authority and by the customer, the print must necessarily be small. So take your reading glasses. People with impaired sight will usually find an assistant or another shopper who will be pleased to help by reading labels. Some stores label areas and shelves clearly; if they do not, point it out to the store supervisor.

Information to look for, apart from the obvious items of type of food, brand and price, are the 'sell-by' date now on most perishable foods and the list of ingredients. As ingredients are usually listed in order of proportion, try to choose those in which salt and sugar are either non-existent or well down the list.

The series of black bars now seen on an increasing array of packaging are primarily designed to be scanned at electronic checkouts, thus speeding up the shopping process, but they are not of immediate interest to the customer.

Paying

Most people still prefer to pay for regular food shopping with cash but this habit is rapidly being replaced by use of cheques, credit cards and stores' own budget accounts. Disabled people may well find these methods advantageous, especially if cash is difficult to see or handle. They also lessen the risk of mugging or petty theft, although it is wise to guard credit cards and cheque books while standing in a queue. If you have a cheque previously made out, do not sign it until the very last minute. But remember that such transactions usually take longer than cash payments and plan accordingly, to avoid delaying other shoppers. Tempers are always shortest in the checkout queues!

Transport

Those who do not have access to a family car, who cannot drive themselves or do not know anyone with whom they can make an arrangement for a regular trip to the shops, should enquire locally about the existence of alternative methods of transport. Several districts offer a variety of means, from voluntary car-pools run by private owner drivers to dial-a-ride services, including mini-buses and fixed, low fare taxi rides for registered disabled people. Some large shopping complexes operate a free hire scheme of wheelchairs for use within the complex. Local libraries, CABs and social service departments will have lists of these facilities.

Home helps are not able to take clients shopping, but will willingly undertake local shopping for essential commodities. Some social services departments supply shopping trolleys to their home helps for this purpose and, in certain circumstances, can supply one of these to a client as an aid to daily living.

In some areas, shopping outings for disabled and elderly people are becoming regular events (usually at Christmas but they can be arranged at other times on request). They are planned ahead and well organised by the local stores with the aid of Age Concern, the police, social service departments and voluntary organisations, and publicised in local shops, libraries and newspapers. Facilities offered include carefree, unhurried and uncrowded shopping at special times, transport to and from shops, wheelchair pushers and other escorts and sometimes even refreshments.

Carrying Shopping

Types of carrying containers vary and must be assessed individually. Baskets and bags on wheels are favoured by many older people but these are not always easy to control and can be a menace to other people. There is a sturdier version which doubles as a portable seat (Figure 6.1).

A four-wheeled plastic mesh pushable basket is now available, although rather expensive. Strong, flat plastic or canvas bags are easier to carry than wide baskets and many people find one of these slung across the body on a strong strap from shoulder to hip is more manageable, leaving both hands free. Some wheelchair users suggest having such a bag fixed between the two handles of the chair at the back, or hanging from a rod fixed between the two arms in the front. Another idea is to stretch a 'bungie' round the back of a wheelchair, round the user's waist and hook the two ends into the handles of a string bag, bearing in mind the fact that the weight of the shopping will affect the wheelchair's centre of gravity (Figure 6.2). It is also possible to hang a bag on the front of a walking frame.

Figure 6.1: Shopping Trolley with Seat

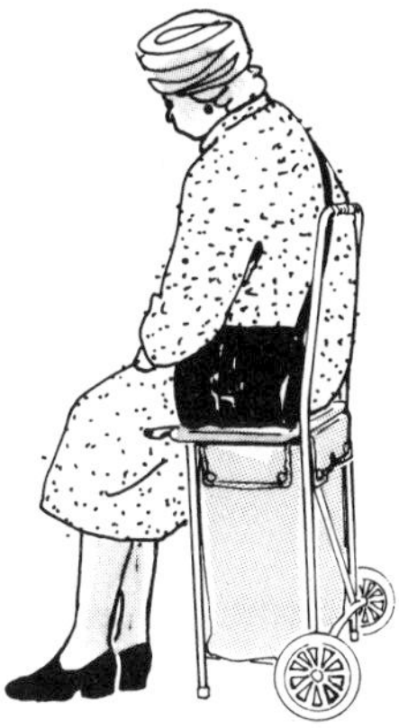

Figure 6.2: Shopping in a Wheelchair with a 'Bungie', Holding the String Bag in Place

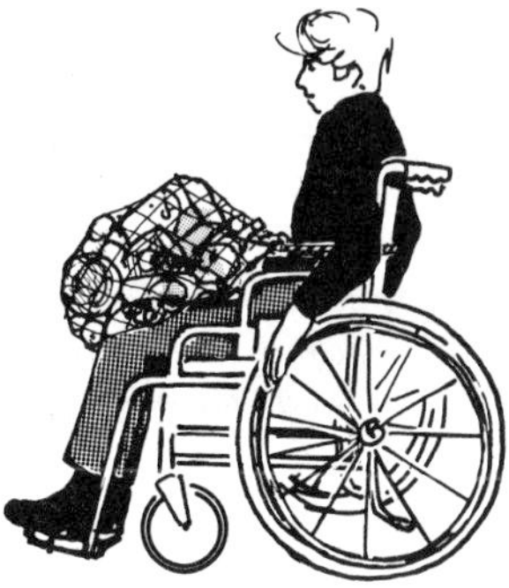

Self-service

Undoubtedly, the biggest single development in food shopping in the last decade has been the expansion in self-service. Even quite small shops have adopted this method of retailing which offers a wider variety of goods and makes more economical use of staff and space. Unfortunately, this can mean inconvenience for the customer and sometimes offers insurmountable obstacles to visually or physically handicapped people. Small, self-service shops often have only narrow spaces between the shelves and turning 'gondolas', making progress difficult for people with sticks and impossible for those in wheelchairs. Other shoppers can also unwittingly cause hazards by blocking the aisles or stepping backwards unexpectedly.

Prices are slightly higher in the small neighbourhood self-service stores, reflecting the higher wholesale prices they have to pay, but this is offset by the convenience of having a nearby local shop open at all hours. It is always worth enquiring whether a local shopkeeper would collect items together for a telephoned order from a disabled person, ready for collection.

Supermarkets

The big supermarket chains have improved their layouts lately for everyone and most of their newer branches offer specially researched facilities for disabled customers. At the time of going to press these include all or most of the following:

1. large adjacent car parks, with specially designated spaces for cars carrying the registered disabled person's orange sticker, as near to the main doors as possible. These may vary slightly to conform with local bye-laws;
2. access to stores on level ground wherever possible, or on a slope, instead of steps;
3. automatic entry and/or exit doors;
4. security turnstiles which can be quickly removed or swung back by an assistant, upon request;
5. wider aisles and circulating areas;
6. clearly labelled departments and displays;
7. new lower-level shopping trolleys, available on request, which can be attached to the front of a wheelchair (Figure 6.3). It does require a certain dexterity to manipulate them! They are also useful for people of short stature, several of whom have suggested borrowing one of the small wheeled trolleys on which shopping baskets are stacked (it would be advisable to ask permission to do this first!);
8. personal assistance for disabled people. All stores welcome requests for help, but do not offer it automatically in case it is resented. So don't be shy! Some stores have staff constantly on the shop floor ready to answer general

Figure 6.3: Low-level Shopping Trolley Attached to Wheelchair

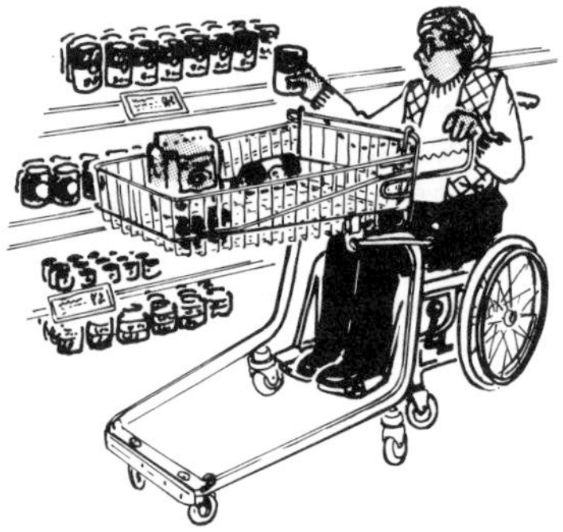

enquiries; others will release an assistant to go round with a customer reading labels, reaching high or low shelves, loading trolleys and finally packing shopping baskets and carrying goods to the customer's car;

9. wider checkouts — each store usually has at least one specially wide checkout, and checkouts where a small number of items can be paid for to avoid waiting. The wide checkout may also be available to others if no disabled people are using it, to avoid wasting staff time;

10. where space and safety permit, seats are sometimes available near the checkouts;

11. toilets, including special ones for disabled people, are becoming more usual in the bigger and newer supermarkets, especially those with restaurants. Some toilets are installed in the car parks;

12. where more than one shopping storey is involved, lifts big enough for wheelchairs are installed;

13. guide dogs are allowed in most supermarkets with their owners, although ordinary dogs are not;

14. first aid is usually available if required.

The foregoing also applies to a number of frozen food supermarkets. The specialised nature of these shops means that sometimes their goods are too heavy or cumbersome to lift out of the freezers. Some stores have a bell at the entrance to summon assistance with negotiating entry, choosing and lifting purchases and carrying them to a vehicle. Some also arrange special evening shopping sessions for groups of disabled people.

If this list sounds too good to be true, be assured that such facilities do exist. If they are not available in your shopping area, do ask for them at the shops you use. It is no good just complaining to neighbours. All stores consulted were emphatic that they are pleased to do what they can to help disabled customers as long as specialised requests do not mitigate against the interests and safety of the community as a whole.

Logical Layout

Shops try to keep commodities arranged in a logical sequence, subject to the space at their disposal and the position of services such as refrigeration. Customers quickly become accustomed to the layout of each shop they visit regularly and take umbrage if the sequence is changed. This can naturally be even more annoying to disabled people, particularly to those with poor sight.

As such an upheaval causes just as much, if not more, trouble for the staff, these changes are not undertaken lightly. If the layout does have to be changed for structural or other major reasons, due notice is given and extra help is available on the shop floor, especially to people who cannot see well.

Hypermarkets

These newer, vast stores selling all kinds of commodities under one roof, are multiplying fast. Inside, most include many of the facilities mentioned for wheelchair users, but they may prove too tiring for many who use sticks and crutches or who cannot see very well, because of the long distances to walk, and the crowds of people.

Human Hazards

The general public has a responsibility to others. Unfortunately, we can all be thoughtless when preoccupied with shopping and all too frequently do not notice the predicament of someone on sticks, in a wheelchair, of short stature or with impaired sight. In spite of all reasonable expectations, the public at large gives little consideration to disabled people, so — BEWARE:

1. shoppers stepping backwards from a window or counter display without looking behind them;
2. groups of people chatting in the aisles, who may suddenly split up;
3. small children who may run amok;
4. prams, pushchairs and shopping baskets on wheels, used as battering rams;
5. people who let swing doors swing back;
6. those agile enough to run up and down steps;
7. people who crowd round the tops and bottoms of escalators;
8. dogs on leads.

Having made these sweeping generalisations, it is only fair to say that the individual is inherently kind and a quiet word or simple request for help or consideration will usually produce the desired result.

Alternative Methods of Shopping

1. Make full use of any delivery services available in your area — very often publicised in local papers or on local radio. Although these services are not as widespread as they used to be, country areas are often reasonably well served by mobile shops selling grocery, greengrocery, bakery, meat, fish and takeaway meals.
2. Milk delivery floats usually carry supplies of fresh, perishable dairy foods and bread.
3. Local markets are friendly places to shop although they do get crowded. Market stall holders will always give cheerful help to wheelchair shoppers.

Permanent covered markets, even if not easy of access, are usually roomy and navigable, once inside.

4. Mail order shopping. Although this method of shopping does not lend itself to regular food shopping, it has a number of advantages for those who cannot get about easily. Goods can be selected at home, and returned if not suitable. Long waits for delivery are a drawback, but usually catalogues are sent well in advance of their relative seasons.

This method of shopping is particularly useful for clothes and household goods, and for presents for birthdays and Christmas, including specialist foods and hampers.

Summary

It is fair to say that conditions for the disabled food shopper have improved considerably within the last decade. The original difficulties have been voiced and many of them overcome, due to the conscience and concern of top management in food retailing, especially in supermarkets. Answers to problems have been found and others are being researched.

Some supermarket chains are considering telephoned orders from a catalogue and a delivery service; some improvement in the design of shopping trolleys might still be made; more handrails, seats and toilets may be desirable. What will the present boom in the use of home computers bring us? Sophisticated shopping no doubt, but perhaps a loss of important personal contact.

It is reasonable to assume that during the next decade automation and electronic devices will continue to improve the lot of everyone who shops. More public awareness of a disabled customer's needs must continue to keep the human angle to the fore.

It is important that economic and ergonomic improvements should favour the community as a whole lest some of the very amenities listed here serve only to segregate disabled people, rather than to integrate them more in day-to-day life.

Whatever happens, help it to happen in your interests by being vocal in a constructive way. If you show courtesy, you will find that other people will respond.

7 Short Cuts in Cooking

Gwen Conacher

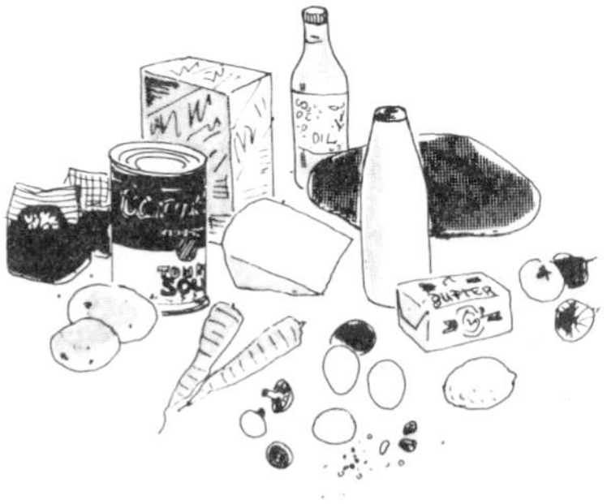

This is not a cookery book, but a book with 'Kitchen sense' in the title would not be complete without some guidelines on easy cooking and a few recipes. What follows is not a catalogue of dull menus, but several simple recipes to encourage you and possibly to set you thinking on new lines. They have all been tested and are liked by those testing and their guests. They are easy and fun to prepare. They will encourage readers to adapt the ideas to their own requirements and to concoct their own specialities along similar lines. Several one-stage mixes are included. Preparation is minimal, yet the finished dishes can look and taste professional. They also heed the nutritional recommendations in Chapter 4.

Convenience foods have an essential place in modern kitchens as they can eliminate a lot of the tedious, repetitive and often difficult preparation. Try to achieve a reasonable balance between prepared convenience foods and market bought fresh produce and utilise a range of canned, dried and frozen foods. A suggested list of basic stores appears on p. 143. Don't be afraid to try new products, either.

The selection of recipes which follows includes main meal dishes for lunch or supper-time, some snacks for the lighter meal of the day (both of which are based mainly on Campbell's condensed soups) and a few teatime bakes which are useful to keep in a tin and enjoy at any time, on your own or with visitors.

Most of the recipes state the number of servings they make, but can be halved or doubled if wished. Quantities are given in metric and imperial measurements. Use whichever scale you prefer, but don't mix the two in one recipe, as they are each worked out proportionally. Always read through the recipes before starting to cook, so you can assemble the necessary ingredients and utensils needed for the job. A list of basic kitchen utensils can be found on p. 145. A simple book rest will make it easier to hold the recipe book open. The recipes marked with an asterisk have been adapted from *Diet 2000*, by Dr. A. Maryon-Davies and Jane Thomas (published by Pan Books).

Main Meal Dishes

Cheesy Potatoes

Ingredients
4 large baked potatoes
150 g (6 oz) Cheddar or Edam cheese, grated
295 g (10.4 oz) can condensed cream of chicken soup
2.5 ml (1/2 tsp) mustard

Method
Cut the potatoes in half lengthways and scoop out about two-thirds of the inside. Mix potato with the cheese, soup, mustard and pepper. Spoon the mixture into the potato shells. Bake in oven at 200 C, 400 F, Gas Mark 6 for 20-25 minutes or reheat under a medium grill for 15-20 minutes. Serves 4.

For a quicker version of this, use prepared instant mashed potato and put the mixture into a heatproof dish. Cook as above.

*Liver Casserole**

Ingredients
450 g (1 lb) lamb's liver
50 g (2 oz) wholemeal breadcrumbs
1 onion, chopped finely or use 1 tbsp dried onion
1 tbsp chopped parsley
1 tsp mixed herbs
Pepper
Grated rind of 1/2 lemon
1 tbsp skimmed milk
225 g (8 oz) can tomatoes, chopped

Method
Preheat the oven to 180°C/350°F/Gas Mark 4. Wash and trim the liver, removing any veins. Cut in slices and place in the bottom of a casserole. Make a stuffing by mixing together the breadcrumbs, onion, parsley, mixed herbs, pepper and lemon rind. Bind together with a little skimmed milk.

Cover the liver with the chopped tomatoes and spread the stuffing mixture on the top. Cover with foil. Cook in the centre of the oven for 30-45 minutes, until the liver is tender, removing the cover for the final 15 minutes to crisp up the top. Serves 4.

*Quick Chicken Curry**

Ingredients
1 medium onion, peeled and chopped
1 tbsp vegetable oil
1 tbsp curry powder
225 g (8 oz) cooked chicken, diced
350 g (14 oz) tin tomatoes
2 tbsp tomato purée
50 g (2 oz) orange lentils
100 g (4 oz) mushrooms

Method
Fry onion in vegetable oil until softened. Add curry powder and fry for a further minute, then add all other ingredients and stir. Bring to the boil, cover and simmer steadily for about 40 minutes. Serves 4.

*Quick Kedgeree**

Ingredients
1 large onion
1 tbsp oil
1 tsp curry powder
450 g (1 lb) cooked rice
200 g (7 oz) tuna, drained and flaked

Method
Slice the onion and fry gently in the oil. Add the curry powder and fry, stirring, for a few minutes. Add the cooked rice and tuna. Stir carefully to distribute the ingredients evenly, producing a warm, golden coloured dish. Do not overcook; the last step is only a mixing and reheating one. Serves 4–6.

Tuna Topped Potatoes

Ingredients
4 large baked potatoes
220 g (8 oz) can tuna
295 g (10.4 oz) can condensed cream of celery soup
100 g (4 oz) grated cheese

Method
Cut the potatoes in half lengthways and scoop out some of the potato (about two-thirds). Drain the tuna and mix it with the soup. Add this mixture to the potato. Pile the mixture into the potatoes and brown under the grill or in the oven. Serves 4.

For a quicker version of this, use prepared instant mashed potato and put the mixture into a heatproof dish. Cook as above.

French Bread Pizzas

Ingredients
1 French loaf
298 g (10.5 oz) condensed cream of tomato soup
3 tomatoes, thinly sliced
150 g (6 oz) cheese, grated
5 ml (1 tsp) mixed herbs
150 g (6 oz) streaky bacon, cut in strips

Method
Cut bread into four pieces, cut in half lengthways. Put on to a baking tray, cut side uppermost. Spoon the tomato soup on to bread, flatten a little but do not spread. Lay tomatoes on soup. Mix cheese and herbs together and sprinkle over tomatoes. Top with bacon. Bake in oven at 200°C, 400°F, Gas Mark 6 for 20-25 minutes until bacon is cooked and cheese is golden brown. Alternatively, put baking tray and pizzas under a medium hot grill for 10-15 minutes. The topping may also be cooked in the oven on top of an easy scone or bread mix. Serves 4.

Wholemeal Pizza

This recipe does not need scales; use instead a 150 g yoghurt pot, or similar size, to measure out ingredients.
Ingredients
Scone base:
$^1/_8$ packet margarine
1 pot wholemeal flour
1 tsp baking powder
1 pot finely chopped onion
2 pots finely grated Cheddar cheese
salt
generous pinch mixed herbs
1 egg
2 tbsp milk

Topping:
4 tomatoes, sliced
3 pots mushrooms, sliced and washed
Generous pinch basil, oregano or mixed herbs
1 pot Cheddar cheese, coarsely grated
Few strips of bacon
Green or black olives, stoned and halved

Method
Place all the ingredients for scone base in a mixing bowl and mix to a fine dough with a wooden spoon. Turn onto a lightly floured board and knead

lightly. Shape into a flat round 20-23 cm (8-9 in) in diameter and place on a greased baking sheet.

Arrange sliced tomatoes and mushrooms on the top. Sprinkle with herbs and cheese and decorate with a lattice of bacon. Place olives in between lattice. Bake for 20-25 minutes at 200°C, 400°F, Gas Mark 6. Serve hot. Serves 2.

Instant Fish Pie

Ingredients
425 g (15 oz) can of mackerel
298 g (10.5 oz) can condensed cream of celery soup
30 ml (2 tbsp) lemon juice
30 ml (2 tbsp) chopped parsley
1 packet instant potato (2-3 servings)

Method
Drain the juice from can of mackerel and remove any large bones. Mix fish with soup, lemon juice and parsley and place mixture in a pie dish. Top with potato, made up as directed on the packet and cook at 190°C, 375°F, Gas Mark 5 for 30-40 minutes. Serves 4.

Salmon and Asparagus Quiche

Ingredients
200 g (8 oz) home-made shortcrust pastry or 350 g (12 oz) ready prepared shortcrust pastry — see recipe for quick pastry with oil on p. 142.

Filling
3 eggs (size 3)
295 g (10.4 oz) can condensed asparagus soup
½ soup can of milk
salt and pepper
198 g (7 oz) can pink salmon *or* 198 g (7 oz) can of drained tuna
1 tbsp chopped fresh parsley
150 g (6 oz) Gouda cheese, grated

Method
Roll out pastry to line a 23 cm (9 in) flan case. Line with foil and put a few bread crusts or baking beans on foil to weigh down pastry base. Bake in oven at 200°C, 400°F, Gas Mark 6 for 20 minutes. Remove foil and bread crusts. For the filling, beat together eggs, soup, milk and seasoning. Drain salmon and remove any bones and skin. Break up the fish roughly, add to filling, with parsley and half of the cheese. Pour filling into flan case making sure it is evenly distributed. Sprinkle remaining cheese on top. Bake in oven at 180°C, 350°F, Gas Mark 4 for 25-30 minutes until filling has set. Serve hot or cold. Serves 6-8.

Souffléd Smoked Salmon

This recipe is easier to make with a food mixer.

Ingredients

15 ml (1 tsp) gelatine
20 ml (4 tsp) water
10 ml (2 tsp) lemon juice
295 g (10.4 oz) can condensed cream of smoked salmon soup
141 g (5 fl.oz) carton soured cream, cottage cheese or quark
milled black pepper
2 egg whites, stiffly beaten
lemon and cucumber slices for garnish

Method

Dissolve the gelatine in the water and lemon juice following instructions on the packet. Combine the soup and soured cream in a large bowl. Pour warmed gelatine quickly into the bowl stirring briskly. Season with pepper. Fold the whisked egg whites into the salmon mixture and pour into a 15 cm (6 in) soufflé type dish. Leave to set in the refrigerator. Do not over-chill. Serve garnished with lemon and cucumber slices. Serves 4.

Salmon Butterflies

Ingredients

350 g (12 oz) pasta butterflies or bows
salt to taste
30 ml (2 tbsp) olive oil
knob of butter
1 onion, peeled and chopped
100 g (4 oz) mushrooms, sliced
295 g (10.4 oz) can condensed cream of smoked salmon soup
150 ml (¼ pt) double cream
pepper to taste
To serve: green salad

Method

Cook pasta in plenty of boiling salted water for 14-15 minutes (or as directed on the packet) until just tender. Heat oil and butter in a pan and gently fry onion for 2-3 minutes. Add mushrooms and continue frying gently for 5-6 minutes until vegetables are tender. Add soup, then stir in the cream and bring to the boil. Drain pasta well and place in a warm serving dish; pour on the sauce, toss well together and sprinkle with plenty of pepper. Serve at once with green salad. Serves 4.

Prawn Stuffed Plaice

Ingredients
125 g (4 oz) shelled prawns
50 g (2 oz) mushrooms, chopped
15 ml (1 tbsp) lemon juice
4 large fillets plaice, skinned
295 g (10.4 oz) can condensed cream of mushroom soup
150 ml (1/4 pt) milk

Method
Mix together prawns, mushrooms and lemon juice. Put a spoonful of prawn mixture on the wide end of skin side of each fillet. Roll up fillets and secure with wooden cocktail sticks if necessary. Place in ovenproof dish.

Cover and cook in oven at 180°C, 350°F, Gas Mark 4 for 20 minutes. Put soup, milk and any remaining stuffing mixture into a saucepan, mix and bring to the boil. Pour over the plaice and serve. Serves 4.

Variations
1. Omit prawns and use either some prepared parsley stuffing mix, or canned mackerel, tuna or cod's roe.
2. Use pieces of any white fish, fresh or frozen and do not stuff and roll.
3. Try the same idea with different condensed soup — chicken, celery or tomato, for instance.
4. Use any cold cooked fish, including smoked fish — heat any flavour soup in a pan, stir in fish. Serve hot with rice.

Light Meal Dishes

Crunchy Chicken Salad

Ingredients
295 g (10.4 oz) can condensed asparagus soup
300 ml (1/2 pt) mayonnaise
salt and pepper
pinch of celery salt
500 g (1 lb) cooked chicken, chopped
small packet of peanuts
lettuce for garnish

Method
Combine soup and mayonnaise, season well and add celery salt. Stir in chicken and half of nuts. Refrigerate. Serve on a bed of lettuce garnished with remaining nuts. Serves 4-6.

Herring Roe Pâté *

No need to spread fat on bread or crispbread when eating this pâté; just eat it by itself, spread thinly, or spread more thickly on hot toast.

Ingredients
50 g (2 oz) margarine
100 g (4 oz) soft herring roes/can of soft cod roe
2 tbsp chopped parsley
1 tbsp lemon juice
pepper

Method
Melt 25 g/1 oz of the margarine in a saucepan. Add the herring roes and fry gently for about 10 minutes. Soften the remaining margarine without melting it. Mash or liquidise the roes. Add the softened margarine, the chopped parsley, lemon juice and pepper. Mix well. Serves 4.

Spanish Omelette *

Ingredients
1 medium onion
1 tbsp oil
100 g (4 oz) mushrooms
450 g (1 lb) cooked potatoes, diced
425 g (15 oz) tin tomatoes, drained and chopped
3 eggs
150 ml (¼ pt) skimmed milk
pepper

Method
Fry the sliced onion in the oil. Add the mushrooms and cook for a few minutes, stirring. Add the potatoes and tomatoes, stir once carefully to distribute.

Beat the eggs, add the skimmed milk and pepper and pour over the vegetables in the pan. Cook slowly, shaking the pan occasionally. When the egg mixture shows signs of being cooked part of the way through, place the pan under the grill to cook the top side until golden brown. Serve the omelette in wedges. Serves 4.

Party Dips

These dips make an easy way to offer light refreshment with drinks or coffee. Make the dips earlier in the day and keep, covered, in the refrigerator. Then serve with small savoury biscuits, fingers of toast or melba toast, and small sticks of celery, cucumber or carrot. These mixtures can also be served spread on biscuits, crispbreads or toast for a more substantial snack. The recipes are based on small 'one-serving' cans, but they can also be made with half a full-size can; use the remainder for 'elevenses'.

Mushroom and Hazelnut Dip

140 g (4.9 oz) can condensed cream of mushroom soup
5 ml (2 tsp) sherry
15 ml (1 tbsp) soured cream
30 ml (2 tbsp) chopped toasted hazelnuts
chopped chives for garnish

Combine all the ingredients together. Serve within 1-2 hours as the hazelnuts become soft if made too long in advance. Garnish with chopped chives before serving.

Curried Chicken Dip

10 ml (2 tsp) lemon juice
1 eating apple
156 g (5½ oz) condensed cream of chicken soup
15 ml (1 tbsp) mango chutney
10 ml (2 tsp) concentrated curry sauce or curry powder
lemon slice for garnish

Mix together lemon juice and grated apple to prevent discoloration. Add the remaining ingredients and mix well. Garnish with lemon twist.

Cheese and Celery Dip

Ingredients
156 g (5½ oz) can condensed cream of celery soup
100 g (4 oz) cheese, grated
2.5 ml (½ tsp) French mustard
salt and pepper

Method
Turn soup into a bowl, add cheese and mustard and mix well. Season to taste. Pour into a serving dish.

Garlic dip

Ingredients
156 g (5½ oz) can condensed cream of mushroom soup
1 clove of garlic, crushed or finely chopped
15 ml (1 tbsp) mayonnaise
two to three pimento-stuffed olives, chopped

Method
Combine soup, garlic and mayonnaise. Leave to stand for 1-2 hours to develop the flavours. Turn into a serving dish and garnish with chopped olives.

Baking — Bread and Cakes

Baking Powder Cob Loaf

Ingredients
250 g (½lb) plain flour — wholemeal
20 ml (4 tsp) baking powder
5 ml (1 tsp) salt
125 ml (¼pt milk)
30 ml (2 tbsp) water

Method
Mix all ingredients in a bowl, as quickly as possible. Form into a smooth ball. Put on floured baking sheet. Bake for 25-30 minutes at 220°C, 425°F, Gas Mark 7.

Easy Wholemeal Bread — Country Style

Ingredients
500 g (1 lb) wholemeal flour or
250 g (½lb) each wholemeal and strong white flour
5 ml (1 tsp) sugar
5 ml (1 tsp) salt
1 packet easy mix yeast
250/375 ml (½/¾pt) warm water

Method
Put flour(s) into a bowl and add salt. Add the yeast. Pour in the warm water and mix well with fork or hand. Put into a greased 1 kg (2 lb) loaf tin and leave to rise until dough reaches the top of the tin. (Put tin into a plastic bag and stand in a warm place.) Bake in a preheated oven for approximately 40-45 minutes, at 220°C, 425°F, Gas Mark 7.

Victoria Sandwich Cake

Ingredients
125 g (4 oz) margarine
125 g (4 oz) castor sugar
2 eggs, size 2
125 g (4 oz) self-raising flour
5 ml spoon (1 tsp) baking powder

Filling
30 ml spoon (2 tbsp) jam
icing or caster sugar, to dredge

All-in-one Method
Grease and flour a 20 cm (8 in) sandwich tin or 2 × 15 cm (6 in) tins. Place all ingredients in a bowl. Beat with a wooden spoon until well mixed (2-3 minutes). (The mixture should be lighter in colour and slightly glossy.) Place mixture in prepared tin(s). Smooth top(s). Bake in a pre-heated oven, for a 20 cm (8 in) tin 35-45 minutes, or 2 × 15 cm (2 × 6 in) tins 25-35 minutes, at 160°C, 325°F, Gas Mark 3. Test before removing from oven. Turn out and cool on a wire tray. When cold, split the 20 cm (8 in) cake. Sandwich the cakes together with jam. Dredge top with caster or icing sugar or decorate with icing.

Fruit Cake

Ingredients
1 large can (or 2 small cans) condensed milk
125 g (5 oz) margarine
750 g (1½ lbs) dried fruit (mixed)
100 g (4 oz) cherries
200 g (8 oz) plain flour
10 ml (2 tsp) mixed spice
5 ml (1 tsp) cinnamon
2 no. 3 eggs
pinch of salt
2.5 ml (½ level tsp) bicarbonate of soda

Method
Grease and line a 18 cm (7 in) round, deep cake tin. Heat oven to 150°C, 300°F, Gas Mark 2. Pour condensed milk into a saucepan. Add margarine, dried fruit and cherries. Place over low heat until milk and margarine have melted; then simmer gently for about five minutes. Remove from heat and set aside to cool.

Pour flour, spices, salt and bicarbonate of soda into a bowl. Add the eggs; add cooled mixture and mix thoroughly. Put into tin and bake on the middle shelf for 1¾-2 hours.

The cake should be well risen, golden brown and feel firm when pressed gently. Leave in the tin for 10 minutes before turning on to a wire rack. Keeps well wrapped in foil or clingfilm.

The next three recipes are simplicity itself, using a 150g yoghurt pot (or similar size) to measure ingredients, instead of scales.

Caribbean Cherry Squares

Ingredients
3/4 packet margarine
2 pots self-raising flour
1 pot castor sugar
2 eggs
1 pot milk
1 pot desiccated coconut
1 pot cherries, halved

Method
Place margarine, flour, sugar, eggs and milk in a bowl with half the pot of coconut. Beat together until smooth. Grease an 18 × 23cm (7 × 9in) baking tin and sprinkle the base with remaining coconut. Spoon mixture on top and spread to the corners. Make rows of cherries in the mixture and bake for 1 hour at 160°C, 325°F, Gas Mark 3. Cool slightly before turning out. Cut into squares when cold.

Quick Fruit Cake

Ingredients
1/2 packet margarine
1 pot soft brown or caster sugar
2 eggs
2 pots self-raising flour
1 pot sultanas, raisins or currants
1 × 450g (1lb) jar mincemeat

Method
Grease a 20cm (8in) deep round cake tin. Place a margarine wrapper in base, foil side down. Mix all ingredients together in a bowl. Beat for 2 minutes or until well mixed. Place in the cake tin and smooth the surface. Bake for about 1 3/4 hours at 160°C, 325°F, Gas Mark 3. Cool slightly before removing from the tin.

Jewel Cake

Ingredients
1/2 packet margarine
1 pot caster sugar
2 eggs
1 pot self-raising flour
1 pot mixed chopped fruit and nuts, for example, mixed peel, angelica, cherries and almonds

Method
Grease a 20cm (8in) round cake tin. Make cake by mixing margarine, sugar, eggs and self-raising flour together in a bowl until smooth. Spoon into tin and bake for 20 minutes at 180°C, 350°F, Gas Mark 4. Sprinkle fruit and nut topping over the cake and return to oven for a further 10-15 minutes. Cool slightly before turning out.

Easy Fruit Loaf

This is also an easy recipe if scales are difficult. Use the same cup for all ingredients.

Ingredients
2 cups self-raising flour
2 large tbsp syrup
1 cup milk and water mixed
½ to ¾ cup fruit (currants, dates, sultanas, apricots, etc.)

Method
Mix well together in a bowl. Put into greased 1kg (2lb) loaf tin and bake for approximately 1½ hours at 160°C, 325°F, Gas Mark 3. Slice and butter when cold.

Small Condensed Milk Cake

Ingredients
25g (1oz) chopped cherries
200g (8oz) mixed, dried fruit
125g (5oz) soft margarine
125g (5oz) plain flour
1 small tin condensed milk with 100ml (¼ pint) water
pinch of salt
2.5ml (½tsp) bicarbonate of soda

Method
Melt the cherries, mixed fruit, soft margarine, and condensed milk and water together, then leave to cool. Add plain flour, pinch of salt and bicarbonate of soda. Turn into a well greased 15cm (6in) tin and bake for 1¼ hours at 160°C, 325°F or Gas Mark 3.

Biscuit Cake (no cooking)

Ingredients
200g (8oz) broken biscuits (crush them in a bag)
50g (2oz) margarine
30ml (2tbsp) golden syrup
45ml (3 level tbsp) cocoa

Method

Melt margarine, syrup and cocoa in a pan over gentle heat. Add crushed crumbs. Mix well. Press into greased tin 20cm (8in) square. Put into cool place or fridge to get cold. Cut into pieces.

Flapjacks

Ingredients

125ml (1/4 pt) corn oil
150g (5oz) demerara sugar
30ml (2tbsp) golden syrup
250g (8oz) rolled oats
pinch of salt

Method

Gently warm the oil, sugar and syrup in a pan and stir oats and salt into them. Press firmly into shallow 20cm (8in) square tin. Bake at 160°C, 325°F, Gas Mark 3 for 25-30 minutes. Leave in tin to cool, then cut into pieces and let them get cold in the tin.

Desserts

Rhubarb Crunch *

Ingredients

450g (1lb) fresh rhubarb
100g (4oz) stoned chopped dates

Topping

25g (1oz) margarine
75g (3oz) wholemeal flour
75g (3oz) rolled oats
25g (1oz) sugar
2tbsp water or orange juice

Method

Clean and slice the rhubarb and add the chopped dates. Mix and place in an ovenproof dish. Rub the margarine into the wholemeal flour, add the oats and sugar, and mix thoroughly. Stir in water so that it is evenly distributed and the mixture has a crumbly texture. Cover the rhubarb with topping and bake at 190°C/375°F Gas Mark 5 for 30-40 minutes. Serves 4.

*Gooseberry Fool**

Ingredients
3 tbsp natural yoghurt
450 g (1 lb) gooseberries
1 egg white
few drops of liquid artificial sweetener

Method
Cook the gooseberries in a very little water until soft, then purée if liked. Stir in the yoghurt and sweetener when the fruit is cool. Beat the egg white and fold into the fruit mixture. Divide into serving dishes and chill. Serves 4.

*Spicy Bread Pudding**

Ingredients
6 slices wholemeal bread
50 g (2 oz) demerara sugar
2 tsp mixed spice
100 g (4 oz) mixed dried fruit
600 ml (1 pt) skimmed milk

Method
Cut the bread into small pieces. Place in a bowl with two-thirds of the sugar, the spice and the fruit. Add the milk and mix thoroughly. Turn into an ovenproof dish and sprinkle with the remaining sugar. Place in a preheated oven, 200°C/400°F/Gas Mark 6, and bake for 30 minutes. Serves 4.

Rice Pudding

Ingredients
40 g (1½ oz) round grain pudding rice
25 g (1 oz) granulated or brown sugar
500 ml (1 pint) milk — fresh, skimmed, evaporated or dried and reconstituted, or use diluted condensed milk and omit sugar
15 g (½ oz) butter or margarine
grated nutmeg — optional for oven version

Method
Wash rice and either:
1. place all ingredients in a saucepan, cover and simmer gently for 1-1¼ hours, stirring occasionally, or;
2. place all ingredients in a greased oven dish and bake for 2 hours at 150°C, 300°F, Gas Mark 2. Sprinkle with nutmeg if liked.

This is a good, versatile dessert. It can be varied as follows:

1. served hot: with stewed or fresh fruit
   with dried fruit cooked in it
   with grated chocolate and/or chopped nuts
2. served cold: as above
   in separate small glass dishes, topped with ice cream and/or fruit purée
   pressed into a ring mould, turned out and served with fruit or a pie-filling in the centre

Miscellaneous

Pastry with Oil

For sweet flan
Short and crumbly. Serve from dish it is baked in.

Ingredients
275g (10oz) plain flour
7.5ml (1½ tsp) caster sugar
120ml (8tbsp) corn oil
60ml (4tbsp) milk
5ml (1 level tsp) salt

Method
Put all the ingredients into a bowl and mix with fork or hand until it forms a ball. Put into a 22.5cm (9in) flan case and push out with hand to cover bottom and sides of the tin.

Alternative (enough for 20cm (8in) diameter flan case)

Ingredients
175g (6oz) plain flour or self-raising flour
75ml (5tbsp) corn oil
4.5ml (3tbsp) water
2.5ml (½ tsp) salt

Method
Put all ingredients into a bowl. Mix with a fork and knead lightly to a manageable dough. Place ball of dough into greased flan tin and press out with fingers.

Basic White Sauce

Ingredients
25g (1oz) margarine

25g (1oz) plain flour
275ml (½ pint) milk (or milk and water, vegetable or bone stock)
salt and pepper

All-in-one Method

1. Place ingredients together in medium-sized saucepan.
2. Stirring continuously over moderate heat, bring to boil and cook for 2-3 minutes until thickened, smooth and glossy.

Soup

Remember that a bowl of soup served on its own, hot *or* cold, makes an easy and appetising meal. For variety, try some of the following ideas, mixing and matching them with different flavours of condensed soup, having followed the diluting and heating instructions on the can.

Soup Serving Suggestions

Sprinkle with freshly chopped green herbs.
Sprinkle with finely chopped hard-boiled egg.
Float with very thin cucumber slices and sprinkle with freshly chopped chives.
Float with croutons and grated Gruyère cheese.
Add 3 tablespoons sherry to soup and sprinkle with freshly chopped parsley.
Sprinkle with freshly grated Parmesan cheese.
Swirl a little single cream into soup.
Sprinkle with chopped crispy bacon.
Float with grated orange peel and chopped chives.
Sprinkle with tiny squares of chopped ham.
Cook with tiny pasta shapes.
Cook with long strands of grated carrot.
Serve with a swirl of mayonnaise.
Float with thinly sliced button mushrooms and sprinkle with chopped parsley.
Swirl with soured cream and sprinkle with a very little grated lemon rind.
Use 3fl.oz (75ml) red or white wine in place of some of the water used for diluting soup. Sprinkle with freshly chopped watercress or parsley.

Standby Stores

Dry Goods

Flour (plain and self-raising, white and wholemeal)
Sugar (brown and white)
Salt
Pepper (white and black)

Mustard
Curry powder or paste
Macaroni or other pasta, wholemeal for preference
Rice (round and long grained)
Dried fat-free milk
Custard powder
Tea/tea bags
Coffee — ground/instant
Vinegar
Cooking oil
Breakfast cereal, or rolled oats for muesli or porridge
Crispbreads
Instant potato powder
Sauce mixes
Beef and chicken stock cubes
Dried onions and vegetables
Dried fruit
Nuts
Jams, marmalade, honey, golden syrup
Bay leaves, cloves, other assorted herbs and spices as liked

Canned Goods
Soups (concentrated or meal-in-one)
Spaghetti sauce (tomato or tomato and mushroom)
Cooking sauces
Evaporated milk and condensed milk
Meat and meat products
Vegetables (tomatoes, new potatoes, butter beans, baked beans, peas)
Fruit, canned in natural fruit juice without sugar
Fish and fish products

Canned and packet foods last a long time, but not for ever. Keep stocks moving. Put new cans or packets at the back of the shelf, bringing old cans forward. A general guide: canned fruits and milk keep in prime condition for about 9-12 months; vegetables — about 2 years; fish in tomato sauce — about 12 months; fish in oil, canned meat — up to 5 years.

Dehydrated foods — vegetables, instant potato, milk powder, coffee powder, etc. — stored in a cool, dry, dark and well ventilated place will keep for up to 12 months unopened.

Basic Freezer Stocks
Breadcrumbs — white and brown (make in blender or processor from crusts of stale bread)
Bread slices (thin) for toasted sandwiches
Bread slices (thicker) for toast

Grated cheese (prepare in blender, or buy from supermarket)
Vegetable purées (made in blender — use in soups)
Stock (made from chicken carcases — use in soups)
Complete plated dinners (plate-up when having a roast joint. Reheat when cooking seems too tiring)
Lemons — whole sliced, grated, or the squeezed juice
Cooked flan cases
Prepared, uncooked pastry (home-made or bought)
Slices of cake, individually wrapped
Loose ice-cubes in a plastic box
Whole (or portions of) cooked dishes to choice

In addition, check weekly that there are adequate stocks of fresh foods in the refrigerator, and replace as necessary, for short-term storage only.

Reminders: milk and milk products, such as skimmed milk, cream, yoghurt
cheese and cheese products, such as cottage cheese
butter, margarine or low-fat spread
eggs
salad ingredients
green and root vegetables
fruit
meat and fish as required

Basic Kitchen Utensils
(Always near to hand)

Drawer
Measuring spoons (a set of British Standard ones)
Tablespoons, forks, knives, teaspoons
Wooden spoons
Spatula
Pastry blender
Chopping knife (sharp), vegetable knife
Vegetable peeler
Can opener (or wall mounted)
Sharp kitchen or needlework scissors
Spike board
Rolling pin
Extras:
Bread knife
Non-slip mat or sponge cloth
Draining spoon
Tongs

Pastry cutters
Whisk
Oven gloves
Asbestos cloth

Cupboard
Mixing bowl (earthenware, plastic or stainless steel)
Basins (graded — plastic)
Measuring jug (in Imperial and Metric)
Sieve
Large and small saucepans (one non-stick)
Frying pan
Chip basket
Chopping board
Extras:
Grater
Cooling rack
Colander
Baking tins
Timer

Appendix I: Sources of Advice and Help

Health and Welfare Services

The Doctor

Whatever problem or query you may have about your health or physical condition, consult your doctor about it before contacting outside organisations, even those specifically connected with your particular situation.

Health Services

These include help given by home nurses, health visitors and occupational and physiotherapists. Ask the doctor about this as you may need his recommendation to obtain their help.

A Home Nursing Service. This can be provided for those who need it because of illness or handicap whether on a temporary or permanent basis. Advice can be given about relevant aids available.

Health Visitors. These are trained nurses, who visit in an advisory capacity only.

Occupational Therapists. In the local authority, they can advise on any appropriate aids that may be necessary to make life easier and more independent, and recommend structural alterations if necessary. A grant towards the cost of these may be available. Each of these can put you in touch with the other and with any alternative help available.

Physiotherapists. These use physical means to treat all forms of injury and diseases to develop and restore the functions of the body. Treatment must be on the recommendation of a doctor and if there is not a domiciliary physiotherapist attached to your local health department, the doctor may arrange for you to attend a hospital department for any treatment he considers necessary.

Social Services

These include social workers, home helps, meals on wheels, laundry service.

Social Workers. These give personal advice and help to anyone in difficulty through illness or stress, and can advise about the appropriate services in the area.

Home Helps. These may be provided for those who need help with main household tasks. A charge is usually made, related to means and based on the number of hours of help given. A doctor's recommendation to obtain this service may be needed, depending on the policy of the local authority.

Laundry Services. These may be provided by the local authority for households where someone is being nursed at home, especially if they are incontinent.

Meals on Wheels. See Chapter 5.

Public Health Department

This department is concerned with the upkeep of health standards in property, so its scope is very wide and includes complaints about rented accommodation and certain stipulations regarding new buildings or extensions. It offers advice on health hazards in the home, for instance, rats, mice, insects, damp, blocked drains, rubbish disposal.

Both the local authority health department and the director of social services can be contacted at your town hall. The appropriate addresses and telephone numbers can also be obtained from the post office, the public library, or the Citizens Advice Bureau.

Other Welfare Organisations (including those specifically concerned with disabled and elderly people)

Age Concern (60 Pitcairn Road, Mitcham CR4 3LL; tel: 01-640 5431). This organisation offers information and advice on all aspects of the welfare of the elderly, and co-ordinates old peoples' welfare committees; can give you the address of your local branch.

British Red Cross (Central Office: 9 Grosvenor Crescent, London SW1; tel: 01-235 5454). Covers many aspects of welfare, nursing and first aid work. It runs clubs and holiday schemes for disabled people and also has a medical loan service enabling those in need to borrow such things as wheelchairs and bedpans through its local branches. It has a catalogue of ideas for aids that can be made at home. There is likely to be a local centre, which can be found in the telephone book.

Citizens' Advice Bureau (National Association: Myddleton House, 115/123 Pentonville Road, London N1 9LZ; tel: 01-833 2181). Deal with any situation needing help, advice, explanation or information — problems concerning family, marriage, social security, legal matters, tax, employment, housing, landlord-and-tenant. Even if the staff cannot answer questions directly, they will be able to put you in contact with someone who can, and all your dealings with them will be kept confidential. The address and telephone number of the nearest bureau can be obtained from the telephone directory or from the public library or the post office, which can also tell you the times the bureau is open. If you are in an area where there is no bureau nearby, the address of the nearest one can be obtained from the information department of the National Association of Citizens' Advice Bureau Council (see p. 148).

Disablement Incomes Group (Advisory Service: Attlee House, 28 Commercial Street, London E1 6LR; tel: 01-247 2128 or 6877). A pressure group whose main aim is to establish a reasonable and national income for disabled people.

The Disabled Living Foundation (380-384 Harrow Road, London W9 2HU; tel: 01-289 6111). Studies all disability with the aim of improving personal and environmental conditions for disabled people. At the London premises there is a comprehensive exhibition of aids, providing a useful centre for anyone to come by appointment to try out equipment. There is also an information service to which anyone can apply for help and advice on any aspect of living with a disability.

Greater London Association for the Disabled (336 Brixton Road, London SW9 7AA; tel: 01-274 0107). Has an information service about local associations and social clubs for disabled people in Greater London. Acts as a pressure group on access and other matters affecting London.

RADAR, The Royal Association for Disability and Rehabilitation (25 Mortimer Street, London W1N 8AB; tel: 01-637 5400). Is concerned with all aspects of physical disability and believes that disabled people should be part of the community and share in all its activities. To achieve this, RADAR campaigns vigorously for the recognition of the needs and rights of disabled people. It provides information and advice to disabled people, their friends and relatives and others in the field of disability, and is particularly active in the following areas: employment, education, access, housing, holidays, social services provision, social security, mobility and general welfare.

RADAR also co-ordinates the efforts of voluntary and statutory bodies working for the welfare and rehabilitation of disabled people. More than 350 of these bodies are members, and to ensure close contact the Association has developed officers in various parts of the country.

Royal Society for the Prevention of Accidents (ROSPA) (Cannon House, The Priory, Queensway, Birmingham B4 6BS; tel: 021-233 2461). Offers advice on all aspects of prevention of accidents and publishes leaflets and booklets at reasonable cost.

Women's Royal Voluntary Service (WRVS) (17 Old Park Lane, London W1Y 4AJ; tel: 01-499 6040). Is concerned with welfare in the widest sense. There are many branches whose addresses and telephone numbers can be found in the relevant phone directories. Apart from organising clubs and other activities for disabled and elderly people they offer personal help including visiting, escort duty, shopping, meals-on-wheels service.

Other Specific Organisations

Arthritis Care, 6 Grosvenor Crescent SW1X 7ER (tel: 01-235 0902)

Association for Spina Bifida and Hydrocephalus have local groups. The central address is 22 Upper Woburn Place, London WC1H 0EP (tel: 01-388 1382)

British Diabetic Association, 10 Queen Anne Street, London W1M 0BD (tel: 01-323 1531)

British Dietetic Association, 103 Daimler House, Paradise Circus, Queensway, Birmingham B1 2BJ (tel: 021-643 5483)

British Epilepsy Association, Crowthorne House, New Wokingham Road, Wokingham, Berkshire RG11 3AY (tel: 0344 773122)

British Migraine Association, Evergreen, 178A High Road, Byfleet, Weybridge, Surrey KT14 7ED (tel: 093 23 52468)

British Polio Fellowship, Bell Close, West End Road, Ruislip, Middlesex (tel: 71 75515)

Centre on Environment for the Handicapped, 35 Great Smith Street, London SW1P 3BJ (tel: 01-222 7980)

Chest and Heart Association, Tavistock House North, Tavistock Square, London WC1H 9JE (tel:01-387 3012)

Colostomy Welfare Group, 38/39 Eccleston Square, London SW1 (tel: 01-828 5175)

Help the Aged, St James Walk, London EC1R 0BE (tel: 01-253 0253)

Ileostomy Association of Great Britain and Northern Ireland, Amblehurst House, Chobham, Woking, Surrey GU24 8PZ (tel: 09905 8277)

Multiple Sclerosis Society of Great Britain, 25 Effie Road, London SW6 1EE (tel: 01-736 6267/78)

Muscular Dystrophy Group of Great Britain, Nattras House, 35 Macaulay Road, London SW4 0QP (tel: 01-720 8055)

National Association for Colitis and Crohn's Disease, 98a London Road, St. Albans, Herts AL1 1NX

National Association for Mental Health (MIND), 22 Harley Street, London W1N 2EG (tel: 01-637 0741)

Parkinson's Disease Society of the UK, 36 Portland Place, London WLN 3DG (tel: 01-323 1174)

Phobics Society, 4 Cheltenham Road, Chorlton-cum-Hardy, Manchester M21 1QN (tel: 061-881 1937)

Royal National Institute for the Blind, 224 Great Portland Street, London W1N 6AA (tel: 01-388 1266)

Royal National Institute for the Deaf, 105 Gower Street, London WC1E 6AH (tel: 01-387 8033)

Scottish Council on Disability, Princes House, 5 Shandwick House, Edinburgh EH2 4RG (tel: 031-229 8632)

Scottish Council for Community and Voluntary Organisations, 18/19 Claremont Crescent, Edinburgh EH7 4QD (tel: 031-556 3882)

Spastics Society, 36 Park Crescent, London W1N 4EQ (tel: 01-636 5020)

Spinal Injuries Association, Yeoman's House, 76 St James's Lane, Muswell Hill, London N10 3DF (tel: 01-444 2121)

Thistle Foundation, 27A Walker Street, Edinburgh EH3 7HX (tel: 031-225 7282)

Appendix II: Addresses of Suppliers

Below are the addresses of suppliers of equipment mentioned in the text.

The Disabled Living Foundation's (DLF) annually updated *Household Equipment* (No. 11A) and *Household Fittings* (No. 11B) *Information Lists* give brief descriptions of many items and services and the names and addresses of suppliers.

AID CALL LTD, 15 Radnor Walk, London SW3 4PB (tel: 01-352 2822)
Portable call system.

ALTERNATIVE PLANS CONTRACTS, 9 Hester Road, London SW11 (tel: 01-228 6460)
Homat Medi kitchen units.

ANYTHING LEFT HANDED, 65 Beak Street, London W1R 3LF (tel: 01-437 3910)

AREMCO, Grove House, Lenham, Kent ME17 2PX (tel: 0622 858502)
Dorsal wrist splint; drinking straw holder clip; ergonomic knife and fork; Manoy beaker; Nelson knife; plastic utensil clip-on; stayput pad; universal ADL cuff.

BAYLIS, T. PO Box 5, Twickenham, Middlesex TW2 6RZ (tel: 01-892 1850).
Orange aids.

BEACON DEVELOPMENTS LTD, 105 Station Road, Ashwell, Baldock, Herts SG7 5LT (tel: 046 274 2214)
U2 form.

BRITISH RED CROSS (see Appendix I)
Cutting aid/bread cutting box; tap turner.

CARTERS, J & A LTD, Alfred Street, Westbury, Wilts BA13 3DZ (tel: 0373 822203)
Mayfair Glideabout; Nelson knife.

CHESTER CARE, 16 Englands Lane, London NW3 4TG (tel: 01-586 2166)
Spring-loaded beater; single-handed tray; tap turner; Twister.

CHUBB FIRE SECURITY LTD, Pyrene House, Sunbury-on-Thames, Middx (tel: 0932 785588)
Fire blanket/fire extinguisher.

CLASSWOOD LTD, Cobham Road, Pershore, Worcs WR10 2DE (tel: 0386 554444)
Turnaid; wooden teapot/kettle tipper.

CLOS-O-MAT (GT BRITAIN) LTD, 2 Brooklands Road, Sale, Cheshire M33 355 (tel: 061-973 6262/4)
Electronic water taps.

CLOTH KITS, Lewes Design Workshops Ltd, 24 High Street, Lewes, East Sussex BN7 2LB (tel: 0273 477111)

CORIAN, Richmond House, 16 Blenheim Terrace, Leeds LS2 9HN (tel: 0532 439651)

Sink moulded with worktop.

DAYS MEDICAL AIDS LTD, Litchard Industrial Estate, Bridgend, Mid Glamorgan CF31 2AL (tel: 0656 60150/57495)

Dycem 'freehand' tray; Dycem plastic material; Nelson knife.

DENROY INTERNATIONAL LTD, 79 Brighton Road, Surbiton, Surrey (tel: 01-399 4151)

Double tier roundabout.

DEPARTMENT STORES

Onion stick; spaghetti tongs.

DROVE PRECISION ENGINEERING, Hargreaves Road, Highfield Industrial Estate North, Eastbourne, Sussex BN23 6QL (tel: 0323 507701)

DPS floating stool.

DYCEM LTD, Ashley Hill Trading Estate, Bristol, Avon BS2 9XS (tel: 0272 559921)

Dycem 'freehand' tray.

ELLARD SLIDING DOOR GEARS LTD, Works Road, Letchworth, Herts SG6 1NN (tel: 046 26 78421)

Sliding windows

ELLIS SON AND PARAMORE LTD, Spring Street Works, Sheffield, South Yorks S3 8PB (tel: 0742 738921)

Hayman perching stool; Belliclamp; bread board with buttering edge.

FRANKE OF SWITZERLAND, UK Sales, Suite 15b, Manchester International Office Centre, Styal Road, Manchester M22 (tel: 061-436 6280)

Sink with strainers.

GILMAX (CATERING): M. Gilbert (Greenford) Ltd, 1109-15 Greenford Road, Greenford, Middx UB6 0EH (tel: 01-864 6566)

Duetto tongs.

HOMECRAFT SUPPLIES LTD, 27 Trinity Road, London SW17 7SF (tel: 01-672 7070)

Amefa knife; Clyde potato peeler; Dycem 'freehand' tray; ergonomic knife and fork; Etwall trolley; long handled opener with steel band; Gripkit handles; Manoy beaker; Nelson knife; Open-all jar opener; plastazote tubing; plug with handle; Rex peeler; Selectacup; Skyline V-grip; spring loaded beater; Twister; wooden teapot/kettle tipper.

HOME NURSING SUPPLIES LTD, Headquarters Road, West Wilts Trading Estate, Westbury, Wilts BA13 4UR (tel: 0373 822313)

Nelson knife.

HUGH STEEPER (ROEHAMPTON) LTD, 237 Roehampton Road, London SW15 4LB (tel: 01-788 8165)

Gripkit handles; Nelson knife.

JAMES SPENCER & CO LTD, Moor Road Works, Headingley, Leeds, West Yorks LS6 4HB (tel: 0532 785837)
Nelson knife.

JONCARE, Radley Road Industrial Estate, Abingdon, Oxon OX14 3RY (tel: 0235 28120)
Cutting aid/bread cutting box; Dycem 'freehand' tray.

LLEWELLYN & CO LTD, Carlton Works, Carlton Street, Liverpool L3 7ED (tel: 051-236 5311)
Bread board with buttering edge; Clyde potato peeler; cutting aid/bread cutting box; Dycem 'freehand' tray; Etwall trolley; Knoon; Knork; Manoy beaker; Mayfair Glideabout; Nelson knife; potato peeler/bean slicer; Skyline V-grip; Turnaid; Twister; window opening device (with lightweight, easy-grip extension handle); wooden teapot/kettle tipper.

MECANAIDS LTD, St Catherine Street, Gloucester, Glos GL1 2BX (tel: 04652 500200)
Easy Reacher reaching aid.

MIDLAND DESIGN ASSOCIATES, 27 Warstone Lane, Hockley, Birmingham, West Midlands B18 6JQ (tel: 021-236 0583)
Swing tray.

MIDLAND ENGINEERING TOOLS CO, Acton Grove, Long Eaton, Notts NG10 1FY (tel: 0602 729888).
Metco Walkabout.

MORSE CONTROLS LTD, Christopher Martin Road, Basildon, Essex SS14 3ES (tel: 0268 22861)
Window opening device (electrically operated).

NICHOLLS AND CLARKE LTD, 3-10 Shoreditch High Street, London E1 6PE (tel: 01-247 5432)
Toggle action taps.

NOTTINGHAM REHAB, 17 Ludlow Hill Road, Melton Road, West Bridgford, Nottingham NG2 6HD (tel: 0602 234251)
Bread board with buttering edge; Clyde potato peeler; Dycem 'freehand' tray; ergonomic knife and fork; Etwall trolley; Gripkit handles; lap tray; Manoy beaker; Nelson knife; plug with grip handle; Selecta-cup; Steelite 80 mugs; Stayput pad; Sunflower kettle tipper; Twister; Turnaid; wooden teapot/kettle tipper.

PAGES, Parke House, 121 Shaftesbury Avenue, London WC2 (tel: 01-379 6334)
Wire coil-spring type whisk (Ritter quirl).

REMAP (Rehabilitation Engineering Movement Advisory Panels), 25 Mortimer Street, London W1N 8AB (tel: 01-637 5400)
Hinged ramp.

REMPLOY, 415 Edgware Road, London NW2 6LR (tel: 01-452 8020)
High stool with back.

ROYAL NATIONAL INSTITUTE FOR THE BLIND (see Appendix I)
Cutting aid/bread cutting box.

SHAVRIN LEVATAP CO, 25 Hatton Garden, London EC1N 8BA (tel: 01-952 8368)
Lever tap.

SHOLLEYS LTD, Crown Works, Crown Close, London E3 2LJ (tel: 01-980 5047)
Plastic mesh basket on wheels.

SISSONS, W AND G LTD, Calver Mill, Calver Bridge, Sheffield, South Yorks S30 1XA (tel: 0433 30791)
Shallow sink.

SML LTD, Bath Place, High Street, Barnet, Herts EN5 5XE (tel: 01-440 6522)
Manoy beaker; Nelson knife; shopping trolley with seat.

TAYLOR AND LAW, 10 Yew Tree Road, London W12 0JT (tel: 01-743 3306)
Clyde potato peeler.

TENDEX PRODUCTS LTD, 121-121A High Street, Edgware, Middlesex (tel: 01-902 7577)
Swivel chair.

TILLING, PETER (PLASTICS) LTD, Building 109, GEC Estate, East Lane, Wembley, Middlesex HA9 7SZ (tel: 01-908 2922)
Long-handled opener with thong.

UNISCAN LTD, Unit 7, Laindon Enterprise Centre, Basildon, Essex SS15 5TE (tel: 0268 419288)
'A' frame.

WAVES, Corscombe, Dorchester, Dorset DT2 0NU (tel: 093-589 248)
Savages Grip clamp.

Appendix III: Further Reading

Chapter 1

British Gas. *Advice for Disabled People* and *Help Yourself to Gas Safety* (leaflets). Gas showrooms or British Gas HQ, 326 High Holborn, London WC1 7PT; tel: 01-242 0789.

Centre on Environment for the Handicapped (1984), *Adapting Kitchens for Disabled People*, CEH, 35 Great Smith Street, London SW1P 3BT; tel: 01-222 7980.

Centre on Environment for the Handicapped. *Windows: Kitchens: Floor Finishes and Surfaces*: Design sheets 2, 4 and 5. CEH (see above)

Cheshire County Council Department of Architecture (1984) *Made to Measure* (3rd edn).

Conran, T. (1982) *The Kitchen Book*, Emblem.

Durward, L. (1983) *Electricity and the Disabled Consumer*, Electricity Consumers' Council, Brook House, 2/16 Torrington Place, London WC1E 7LL.

Electricity Council. *Lighting and Low Vision* (jointly with Partially Sighted Society), *Making Life Easier for Disabled People, Safety in the Home* and *Guidelines to Kitchen Planning* (leaflets). Electricity Council, 30 Millbank, London SW1P 4RD.

Equipment for the Disabled. (1981) *Home Management* (5th edn, 1986) *Housing and Furniture* (5th edn) Equipment for the Disabled, Mary Marlborough Lodge, Nuffield Orthopaedic Centre, Headington, Oxford OX3 7LD.

Ford, M. and Heshel, T. (1982) *In Touch: Aids and Services for Blind and Partially Sighted People* (3rd edn) BBC, 35 Marylebone High Street, London W1M 4AA.

Foott, S. (1977) *Handicapped at Home*, Design Council.

Goldsmith, S. (1984) *Designing for the Disabled* (3rd edn, revised) RIBA Publications.

Harpin, P. *With a Little Help*, Muscular Dystrophy Group of Great Britain, Nattras House, 35 Macaulay Road, London SW4 0QP.

Hayle, G. (1983) *The New Source Book for the Disabled*, Heinemann.

Hunt, J. and Hoyes, L. (1980) *Housing the Disabled*, Torfaen Borough Council.

Jay, P. (1984) *Coping with Disability*, Disabled Living Foundation.

— (1985) *Help Yourselves*, Ian Henry.

Lockhart, T. (1981) *Housing Adaptations for Disabled People*, Disabled Living Foundation, pp. 29-35.

National Building Agency. (1978) *The Disabled in Rehabilitated Housing*, NBC.

National Gas Consumers' Council. *Gas Consumers' Council's Guide.* Guide to the services and benefits available for elderly and disabled people from local gas showrooms, or the National Gas Consumers' Council, 4th Floor, 162 Regent Street, London W1R 5TB.

Penton, J. and Barlow, A. (1980) *A Handbook of Housing for Disabled People* (2nd edn), London Housing Consortium West Group.

Royal National Institute for the Blind. *Running Your Own Home*, 224 Great Portland Street, London W1N 6AA.

'Update: domestic kitchen design'. (1984) *Architects Journal*, 3 October/7 November, p.69.

Walter, F. (1968) *An Introduction to Domestic Design for the Disabled*, Disabled Living Foundation, pp. 13-17.

Chapter 2

British Gas. *Advice for Senior Citizens, Advice for Disabled People, Helpfuel Services from the Gas People, Help Yourself to Gas Safety.* Gas showrooms or British Gas HQ, 326 High Holborn, London WC1V 7PT.

Cox, H.M. (1977) *Cooking Under Pressure*, Faber and Faber.

Electricity Council. *Information sheets* on all domestic electric appliances mentioned in the text are available (free) on request from Electricity Board shops, or post free from Publications Dept, The Electricity Council, 30 Millbank, London SW1P 4RD.

Electricity Council. *Electricity and You* (leaflets on use of electricity in the home). Available (free) on request from Electricity Board shops, or post free from Publications Dept, The Electricity Council, 30 Millbank, London SW1P 4RD.

Electricity Council. *Food Freezing at Home* (booklet in Braille). Available from RNIB (see Appendix I).

Jay, P. (1972) *Cleaning Equipment: A Guide to Choosing Domestic Cleaning Equipment*, Disabled Living Foundation.

Ministry of Agriculture. *An ABC of Home Freezing*, Bulletin 214, HMSO.

Webb, J. (1978) *The Microwave Cookbook*, Forbes Publications.

Webb, J.M. and Conacher, G. (1980) *Microwave Cooking at Home*, Electricity Council (a general guide not a cookery book).

RNIB. *Microwave Instructions and Recipes* (for details of microwave oven instructions and recipe books in Braille and a tape, contact Customer Liaison Officer, RNIB; see Appendix I).

Journals

WHICH? Journal of the Consumers' Association, 14 Buckingham Street,

London WC2N 6DS. Monthly. Includes reports of comparative testing of household and kitchen equipment. Most public libraries hold back copies and indexes.

Journal Articles

'Scaling Down: GHI Thinks Small about Big Essential Equipment', *Good Housekeeping*, March 1984, pp. 76-81.

Chapter 3

Ansell, B and Lowton, S. (1985) *Your Home and Your Rheumatism*, Arthritis and Rheumatism Council.

Bradshaw, E. (1984) 'Evaluation of kitchen and household equipment' (DHSS Aids Assessment Programme), *Demonstration Centres in Rehabilitation Newsletter*, autumn, pp. 11-17.

— *Food Preparation Aids for Rheumatoid Arthritis Patients* (Parts 1 and 2a). From DHSS Store, Health Publications Unit, No 2 Site, Manchester Road, Heywood, Lancs 0L10 2PZ.

Darnborough, A. and Kinrade, D. (1984) *Directory for the Disabled* (4th edn), Woodhead Faulkner.

Disabled Living Foundation (1969) *Disabled Housewives in Their Kitchens: A Series of One-day Conferences*, Disabled Living Foundation.

Equipment for the Disabled. (1981) *Home Management* (5th edn), Equipment for the Disabled, Mary Marlborough Lodge, Nuffield Orthopaedic Centre, Headington, Oxford OX3 7LD.

Foott, S. (ed.) (1976) *The Disabled Schoolchild and Kitchen Sense.* Disabled Living Foundation.

— (1977) *Handicapped at Home*, Design Council.

Hale, S. (ed.) (1983) *The New Source Book for the Disabled*, Heinemann.

Howie, P.M. (1967) *A Pilot Study of Disabled Housewives in Their Kitchens*, Disabled Living Foundation.

Jay, P. (1984) *Coping with Disability*, Disabled Living Foundation.

— (1985) *Help Yourselves*, Ian Henry.

McIntosh, R. *Food Preparation Aids for Those With Neurological Conditions*, DHSS Aids Assessment Programmes, DHSS Store, Health Publications Unit, No 2 Site, Manchester Road, Heywood, Lancs 0L10 2PZ.

Chapter 4

Davies, L. (1972) *Easy Cooking for One or Two*, Penguin.

— (1979) *More Easy Cooking for One or Two*, Penguin.

Morley, G, (1969) *Good Food on a Budget*, Penguin.

Sainsbury's Food Guides: *Balancing your Diet; Cooking Made Easy for Disabled People; Food for One.* Sainsbury's shops or by post from Public Relations Dept, J. Sainsbury plc, Stamford House, Stamford Street, London SE1 9LL.

Thomas, J. and Maryon-Davis, A. (1984) *Diet 2000*, Pan.

Chapter 7

Atterbury, S. *Leave It To Cook*, Penguin.

Berry, M. *One Pot Cookery*, Hamlyn Publishing Group.

— *Popular Freezer Cookery*, Octopus Books.

Campbell, C. *Cooking For a Busy Day*, Campbells Soups Ltd, Kings Lynn, Norfolk.

Chetwood, D. *Look and Cook* Large print recipe cards. Mrs D. Chetwood, 9 Newlands Road, Sidmouth, Devon EX10 9NL.

Collins, V. *The Complete Microwave Cookbook*, David and Charles.

Cox, H.M. *The Multi Cooker Book*, Faber and Faber.

Emmerson, M. *The Microwave Cookery Course*, Good Housekeeping.

Family Circle *Mixer Cook Book*, Family Circle Books, London WC1N 3QJ (by post only).

Good Housekeeping Institute *Home Freezer Cookbook*, Ebury Press.

Homepride *Book of Home Baking*, Spectator Publications.

Innes, J. *Pauper's Cook Book*, Penguin.

Kenwood. *The Kenwood Blender Book*, Kenwood.

— *The Kenwood Mixer Book*, Kenwood.

Klinger, J.L. *et al. Mealtime Manual for the Aged and Handicapped*, New York University Medical Center, Institute of Rehabilitation Medicine.

Llewellyn, A. *The RNC Cook Book*, Royal National College for the Visually Handicapped, 1984 (see also cassette section).

Marshall, R.M. *My Cook Book*, BIMH Publications (British Institute of Mental Handicap, Wolverhampton Road, Kidderminster, Worcs DY10 3PP).

Morris, M. *The Large Print Cook Book*, Chivers Lythway.

Norwak, M. *Beginners' Guide to Food Freezing*, Pelham Books.

Page, D. *Slow Cooking Properly Explained*, Paperfronts, Elliot Right Way Books, Kingswood, Surrey.

Reekie, J. *Easy Does It Cookbook*, Quiller Press (distributed by Arrow Books).

RNIB. *A Feeling For Food: Cookery Books for Visually Handicapped People* (for details contact customer liaison officer, RNIB; see Appendix I).

Smith, D. *How to Cheat at Cooking*, Coronet.

Cookery Books on Cassette

Davies, L. *Easy Cooking for One or Two.* Send 2 blank C60 cassettes with addressed label for return to: *Mrs Audrey Artus, ADA, 12 Renhold Road, Wilden, Bedford (tel: 0234 771693).*

Leeming, C. Cassette of recipes for blind cooks. Send one blank C60 cassette with addressed label for return to: *Mrs Audrey Artus, ADA, 12 Renhold Road, Wilden, Bedford (tel: 0234 771693).*

Patton, M. Collection of recipes on tape. These cost £1 per cassette from *Nigel Verbeek of Soundaround Magazine, 61 Church Road, Barnes, London SW13 (tel: 01-741 3332).*

Stephenson, V. *Grow and Cook.* Send 3 blank C60 cassettes to *Mrs Audrey Artus, ADA, 12 Renhold Road, Wilden, Bedford (tel: 0234 771693).*

Various voluntary societies record material on request for people in their area. The addresses can be obtained from RNIB.

Several reading services will also record recipes:

Mrs Audrey Artus, 12 Renhold Road, Wilden, Beford (tel: 0234 771693).

George Causey, Agorita, 31 Fortescue Road, Paignton, Devon TQ3 2BY (tel: 0803 522873).

Glasgow Playback Service for the Blind have a tape of recipes suitable for the more experienced cooks and one on yeast cookery. Enquiries to: 276 St Vincent Street, Glasgow G2 5RP (tel: 041-248 5811).

Monument Tape Service 'Townsend', Thorne St Margaret, Wellington, Somerset TA21 OEQ (tel: 0823 672104).

Tape Recording Service for the Blind, 48 Fairfax Road, Farnborough, Hants GU14 8JP (tel: 0252 47943).

Tarporley Recording Centre, 79 High Street, Tarporley, Cheshire (tel: 08293 2115).

Local Talking Newspapers can often help, or contact: Talking Newspaper Association of the UK (Secretary) Mr Cyril Cox, 130 Chester Road, Watford, Herts (tel: 01-954 6111).

Index

accidents 20, 125
activity zones/sequences 7
advice, sources 147-51
Age Concern 148
Aged: Help the Aged 150
alcohol 110
Arthritis Care 150
Association for Spina Bifida and
  Hydrocephalus 150
autochop 71

baking 82
  bread and cake recipes 136-40
  tins, greasing 78
beating, whisking 75, 77
bending 88
blenders 46
Blind, Royal National Institute for 150
body weight, adjustment 111-12
book lists (bibliography) 156-60
bottle openers 66
bowls, types 76
bread, baking recipes 136
  cutting and spreading 72-3
British Diabetic Association 150
British Dietetic Association 150
British Electrotechnical Approvals
  Board (BEAB) 32
British Epilepsy Association 150
British Migraine Association 150
British Polio Fellowship 150
British Red Cross 148
British Standard on housing design for
  disabled people 1, 3, 4

cake making 74-8
cakes, baking recipes 136
calcium, sources in food 109
can openers, electric 47
  manual 66, 68
carbohydrate 108
carrying 90-4
carving 95
  knives, electric 47
ceiling finishes 16
Centre on Environment for the
  Handicapped 150
chairs 58
Chest and Heart Association 150
chopping 70-3
circuit breakers 17
Citizens' Advice Bureaux 148
clamps 64, 67
cleaning 102-4
Clyde potato peeler 70
coffee making and serving 44, 101
Colostomy Welfare Group 150
colour 61
Community and Voluntary
  Organisations, Scottish Council for
  151
condensation 16
continental cookers 30
convenience foods 59, 127
cookers, built-in or 'split level' 30
  choice 36
  cleaning 26, 31
  continental 30
  electric 27-30
    controls 29
    grill 29
    hob 28
    oven 29
    safety and service 32
  free-standing 24
  full-size 22
  gas 23-7
    hob 25
    oven 25
    safety and service 33-4
    special controls 26
  height 13
  hoods 19
  liquefied petroleum gas (LPG) 27
  microwave 40, 60
  multi-purpose 39
  oven temperature equivalents 35
  pressure 80
  running costs 35
  safety and service 32-4
  table top 37
cooking

short cuts 127-46
light meal dishes 133-4
main meal dishes 128-33
miscellaneous 142-3
slow 57
stabilising pans on hob 79
using hob 79
utensils, choice 80
corkscrews 66
cream cheese makers 47
cupboards 14, 15
contents 145
doors, shelved 14
cups 99
cutlery 95-8
one-handed 96
cutting 70-2

day centres, eating at 115
Deaf, Royal National Institute for 151
deep-fat fryers 39
design of kitchen 1-21
desserts, recipes 140-2
Diabetic Association, British 150
Dietetic Association, British 150
Disability and Rehabilitation, Royal Association for (RADAR) 149
Disability, Scottish Council on 151
Disabled, Greater London Association for 149
Disabled Living Foundation 149
Disablement Incomes Group 149
dishwashers 52
doors, removal 6, 16, 63
draining boards 10, 13
drawers 16, 63
drinking devices 99-100
Dux knife 96
Dycem freehand tray 93
slip-resistant material 64

eating
devices 95-8
healthy 106-12
in company 113-17
local authority arrangements 114
out 115-17
eggs, boiling 47, 82
breaking and separating 78
electric
can openers 47
cookers 27-30 *see also* cookers, electric kettles 43
plugs 18, 88
electricity
socket outlets 17, 18, 88
wiring regulations 18
energy conservation 57
Epilepsy Association, British 150
equipment 22-55
choice 60-2
Etwall trolley 91

fan, extractor 19
'fast food' bars 115
fat, sources in food 108
fatigue, avoidance 60
fibre, dietetic 108
fire blankets 20
extinguishers 20
floor
cleaning 89, 103
finishes 16
flour handling 74-5
food, blenders 46
labelling and storage 62
mixers 46
preparation, holding and steadying 64
processors 46
standby stores 143
stored ready prepared 57
trays, heated 45
trolleys, heated 45
foods, 'convenience' 59, 127
freezers 50-2, 60
basic stock 144
use 85
fruit peeling 74
stoning 74
fryers, deep-fat 39
frying precautions 81
fuse box 17

gas cookers 23-7 *see also* cookers, gas
leaks 34
supply 17
gloves, oven 83
grants for kitchen design and improvement 1, 4
grating 73
greasing tins 78
Greater London Association for the Disabled 149
grills 24, 29
contact 37

Handicapped, Centre on Environment

for 150
handles 15
  enlarging 95
Hayman perching stool 58
health and welfare services 147-51
  visitor 147
Heart: Chest and Heart Association 150
heating 19
heights of working surfaces 4, 12
help, sources 147-51
Help the Aged 150
hobs 25, 28, 79
holding aids 64
home help 148
  nursing service 147
housing, adaptation for handicapped 4
    design for disabled, British Standard 1, 3, 4
Hydrocephalus, Association for Spina Bifida and 150

ice cream makers 47
Ileostomy Association 150
internal depth of kitchen units for wheelchair users 10
iron, sources in food 109
irons, electric 54

jar openers 65

kettles, electric 43
key-opening cans 68
kitchen, cleaning 102
  contents 5
  design 1-21
    British Standard
      recommendations 1,3
    local authority grant 1, 4
  development 2
  equipment 22-55
    choice 60-2
  finishes 16
  floor space 3
  planning (layout) 5-7
  safety and security 20
  storage facilities 14-16
  taps 11, 86
  units, design 4
    standard dimensions 7-9
  utensils, basic 145-6
knife, electric 47
  Nelson 96-7
knives 70

labelling food 62
laundry appliances 53-4
  services 148
lifting and carrying 89-94
light dishes 133-4
lighters for ovens 82
lighting 18
liquids, body requirements 110
local authority grants for kitchen design and improvement 1, 4
LPG cookers 27
luncheon clubs 114

mail order shopping 126
main dishes 128-33
Manoy beaker 99
mats, non-slip 64
Mayfair Glideabout 58-9
meals
  on wheels 114
  serving 94-5
meat cutting and mincing 73
menus, planning 57
Metco Walkabout 92
meters, accessibility 17
microwave cookers 40, 60
Migraine Association, British 150
mincers 73
MIND (National Association for Mental Health) 150
mineral salts in food 109
mirror, cooking aid 79
mixing, beating 75, 76, 77
  bowls 76
mobility around kitchen 88-94
mops 89
mugs 99
Multiple Sclerosis Society 150
Muscular Dystrophy Group 150

National Association for Colitis and Crohn's Disease 150
National Association for Mental Health (MIND) 150
Nelson knife/fork 96-7
non-slip material 64
nutrients in food 107-10

occupational therapist 147
one-handed baking 82
  bread spreading 73
  cake making 75
  can opening 47

cutlery 96-7
extracting from oven 83
mixing/beating 77
trays 92
washing up 87
onion stick 71
openers (cans, bottles, jars) 65-8
Orange Aids System 64
oven 25, 29
cleaning 26, 31
extracting dishes 83
gloves 83-4
lighting 82
microwave 40-2
temperature equivalents 35
overweight, management 111

paint, choice 16
pan guard 79
pans, choice 79-80
Parkinson's Disease Society 150
party dips 134-6
pastry making 74-8
peeling and peelers 68-70
Phobics Society 150
physiotherapist 147
pick-up sticks 89
planning, kitchen 5-7
menus 57
shopping 57
plates 97-8
Polio Fellowship, British 150
potato peeling 68
pots, slow-cooking 39-40
pouring 74
power plugs 18, 88
pressure cookers 80
protein, sources 108
Public Health Departments 148
pull-out boards 13
pull-out trays 14

RADAR 149
ramps 83, 91
reaching and bending 88
recipes 128-43
refrigerators 48-50, 51, 84-5
food storage in 50
refuse disposal 11, 20, 102
roasting 82-3
Royal Association for Disability and Rehabilitation (RADAR) 149
Royal National Institute for the Blind 150
Royal National Institute for the Deaf 151
Royal Society for the Prevention of Accidents (ROSPA) 149

safety 20, 34, 91
salt in diet 109
sandwich toasters 38
Savage's grip clamp 68
scales 74-5
scissors 71
Scottish Council for Community and Voluntary Organisations 151
Scottish Council on Disability 151
security in kitchen 20
serving meals 94-5
shelves, adjustable 9, 15
shopping 118-26
alternative methods 125
budgeting 120
carrying 121
hazards 125
hypermarkets 125
in-store information 120
logical layout 124
paying 121
planning 57, 119
self-service 122
supermarkets 123
transport to shops 121
when to shop 119
sieving 75
sinks 10, 86
cleaning 104
skin disorders, dietetic treatment 112
slicing 70
slip-resistant material 64
snacks 133
social services 147
social worker 147
soups, serving suggestions 143
Spastics Society 151
spike board 47, 70
Spina Bifida, Association for 150
Spinal Injuries Association 151
spoons 96
spreading 73
steamers 80
stirring 79
stools 58
storage facilities 14-16
food 62-3
straws 100

suction cups, pads 64, 75, 79
supermarkets 123
suppliers, addresses of 152-5
switches 18-19, 88

table cookers 37
tables, cantilever 58
take-home meals 115
taps 9, 11, 86
  turning aids 86
tea making and serving 44, 100-1
temperature (oven) equivalents 35
Thistle Foundation 151
tin openers, electric 47
toaster ovens 38
toasters 37, 38
trays 92
  for wheelchairs 58, 93
  heated 45
  one-handed 92
tremor, cutlery for 98
trolleys 83, 91
tumble dryers 54

underweight, management 112
utensils, kitchen, basic 145-6

vegetables, straining 73
  peeling 68
  racks 63
ventilation 19
vitamins in food 108

walls, finishes 16
washing machines, automatic 53
washing-up machines 52, 87
waste disposal 11, 20, 102
water, boiling 100
  body requirements 110
  heaters 43-4
  supply 17
  taps 9, 11, 86
weighing 74
wheelchair and mobility housing 4
  in kitchen 2
  internal depth of kitchen units for users 10
whisking 77
window, cleaning 105
  opening devices 19
  siting 3
wine bottle openers 66
woks 81
Women's Royal Voluntary Service (WRVS) 150
working comfort 57
  heights 4, 12, 57
worktops 12
wrists, stiff, cutlery for 98

yoghurt makers 47

	DATE DUE		